Dental Foundation Training

THE ESSENTIAL HANDBOOK FOR FOUNDATION DENTISTS

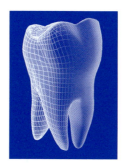

AMIT RAI

General Dental Practitioner
Dental Foundation Training Programme Director
Advisor on Dental Education to the General Dental Council

Foreword by

RAJ RATTAN MBE

BDS MFGDP FFGDP DipMDE
Strategic Associate Dean, London Deanery

Radcliffe Publishing
London • New York

Radcliffe Publishing Ltd
St Mark's House
Shepherdess Walk
London N1 7BQ
United Kingdom

www.radcliffehealth.com

British Library Cataloguing in Publication Data

A catalogue record for this book is available from the British Library.

ISBN-13: 978 184619 997 4

The paper used for the text pages of this book
is FSC® certified. FSC (The Forest Stewardship
Council®) is an international network to promote
responsible management of the world's forests.

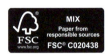

Typeset by Darkriver Design, Auckland, New Zealand
Printed and bound by Hobbs the Printers, Totton, Hants, UK

Contents

Foreword by Raj Rattan

The Greek philosopher Heraclitus wrote that 'No man ever steps in the same river twice, for it's not the same river and he's not the same man'. He was referring to the constant change in the river as it flows so changing from one moment to the next. The same change affects the man. We may do something repeatedly, but each event is subtly different and we become what we are as a result of those experiences.

The statement is true of the world around us and it is certainly true of Dental Foundation Training. Dentistry in the NHS has changed since the early days of vocational training and is set to change again as the Government finalises its proposals for a new dental contract. At the time of writing, we do not have the details of those proposals but we are able to make some assumptions through inductive and deductive reasoning. Some may say that to publish a book in this climate is risky because it may become out of date. That may be true of some of the terminology and career development opportunities, but the essence of this text is about education and the ethos of education shall always remain the same.

Amit has distilled that ethos and used his personal experience as a Trainee, Trainer and Programme Director to inform the text. The writing is a blend of relevant educational theory and practical advice in the context of general dental practice. Importantly, the author highlights the risks in everyday practice; DF Trainees face a challenging post-qualification professional environment where the incidence of dento-legal cases is at an all-time high. Patient complaints and the threat of litigation undermine confidence and can stymie in-practice education, stalling the educational journey. The learner becomes fearful and the reflective learning cycle delivers the wrong conclusion. As Heraclitus put it, 'The road up and the road down are the same thing.'

This book is written from a practical perspective and the author's experience in the field is clearly to be seen. It is a very readable text and Amit has covered all the essential areas to facilitate what was in the early years of vocational training described as a sheltered entry into general dental practice.

Raj Rattan MBE
BDS MFGDP FFGDP DipMDE
Strategic Associate Dean, London
January 2014

Preface

Over the last decade I have been fortunate enough to encounter the full Foundation Training experience. This experience started for me as a fresh-faced vocational dental practitioner, to being appointed as a trainer on the same scheme, right through to my role as a Programme Director, where I went on to establish the Central London Dental Foundation Training scheme. My Programme Director role involved leading a Training the Trainer programme in which I came to appreciate the common challenges encountered by trainers. These collective experiences have helped to shape the content of this book.

This is a really exciting time for new entrants into the profession, and the aim of writing this guide is to help Foundation Dentists get the most out of the year ahead by helping to promote a deeper understanding of Foundation Training. The content that follows is explicit about the ingredients of a successful Foundation Training experience but not about the flavour of that experience, which is very much created by individual training practices and schemes.

This guide is mainly aimed at the Foundation Dentist, as reflected in the style of narration, although it may also prove useful to those undertaking Competency Assessment (FT equivalence) and key stakeholders of Foundation Training. What I hope comes clearly across from the pages that follow is that, to quote George Bernard Shaw (1856–1950), I am:

> a fellow traveler [*sic*] of whom you asked the way. I pointed ahead – ahead of myself as well as you.

Amit Rai
January 2014

About the author

Amit Rai is a general dental practitioner and graduate of the University of Manchester. He is a past Educational Supervisor and Dental Foundation Training Programme Director. Amit acts as an advisor to the Chief Executive of the General Dental Council on matters of Dental Education and works for NHS England both as a dental advisor and as the appointed Chair of a Dental Local Professional Network. He is a fellow of the Higher Education Academy, the Academy of Medical Educators and the Pierre Fauchard Academy. Amit is an accredited Expert Witness in the field of general dental practice, independently considering dental negligence claims. He acts as both an examiner and question writer for the National Examining Board for Dental Nurses. Amit is also an award-winning writer as recognised by the British Dental Editors Forum in 2013.

Acknowledgements

Foundation Training is very much team driven, continuing to evolve ever since its origin in 1977. I feel that Foundation Training would not be the accomplished programme that we see today were it not for the commitment of all Educational Supervisors (trainers), Programme Directors, Associate Deans and Deans, both past and present.

All of the Foundation Dentists that I have had the privilege of guiding – they are my inspiration for writing this book, stemming from the simple desire to ensure that they are well supported, which in turn benefits the patients at the end of this entire process. My gratitude to COPDEND (the UK Committee of Postgraduate Dental Deans and Directors) and to Mike Kelly, who was my Vocational Training Adviser not once but twice within the UK's earliest founded Vocational Training scheme – first, when I was a Vocational Dental Practitioner, and, second, in my career as a trainer. I owe Mike a debt of gratitude for making me see the difference between being a teacher and an educator.

I am grateful to Raj Rattan for his endless support and encouragement, particularly when I was starting out as a Programme Director. Mandy Platts, Andrew Wilson and Robert Clarke have fuelled my understanding of the application of medical education and some of the content of this book is based on what I have gleaned by facilitating alongside them. Writing this book undoubtedly impinged upon my weekends, which affected nobody more so than my wife, who had to entertain our Airedale Terrier puppy on her own during his 'rebellious period'. I will now have to think of another excuse not to walk the dog.

My brother who has been, and remains, an inspiration to me – he is the reason why I entered the profession.

Last but not least, I wish to note the opportunity given to me by Radcliffe Publishing in offering to publish my very first book. They have been very patient in waiting for me to become available – I certainly hope it was worth the wait.

This book is dedicated to my parents.

What is Foundation Training?

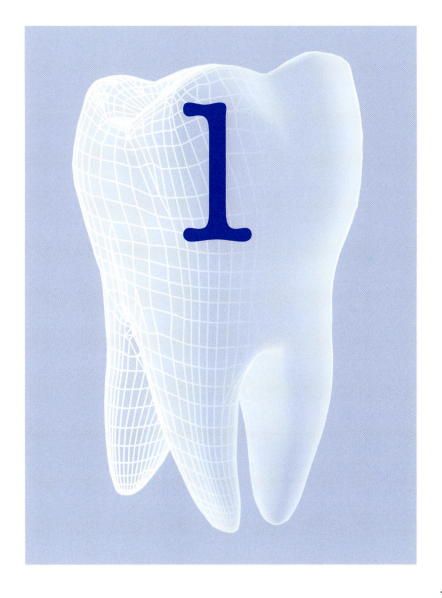

Foundation Training is the training programme that most[1] UK-qualified dentists must complete to gain inclusion as a dental performer onto a UK NHS dental performers list in order to perform National Health Service (NHS) primary dental services without supervision. The programme enables the practice of dentistry within a supervised setting in general dental practice.

More specifically, Foundation Training is defined[2] as:

> a relevant period of employment during which a dental practitioner is employed under a contract of service by an approved trainer to provide a wide range of dental care and treatment and to attend such study days as that contract provides.

This relevant period of employment is either of 1 year's full-time employment or an equivalent period of part-time employment. At the time of writing there are approximately 78 FT schemes, located in thirteen regions across England, Wales and Northern Ireland. For the majority of these schemes the FT programme commences on a fixed date in September each year[3] and for two schemes the start date is in March. The number of schemes is subject to change.

The General Dental Council (GDC) has endorsed the arrangement of Foundation Training (FT) which *'allows a gradual and controlled transition from the shelter of undergraduate education to unsupervised practise'*.[4]

The NHS (Performers Lists) (England) Regulations 2013 outlines the aims and objectives of FT as:[5]

> enhancing clinical and administrative competence and promoting high standards through relevant postgraduate training.

And in particular to:[6]

> a) enable the dental practitioner to practise and improve the dental practitioner's skills;

---

1   Unless the dental practitioner is exempt from the requirement to undertake foundation training as outlined in The NHS (Performers Lists) (England) Regulations 2013, p. 3, ¶34 (4).
2   The NHS (Performers Lists) (England) Regulations 2013, p. 3, ¶30 (1).
3   www.copdend.org/content.aspx?Group=press%20releases&Page=press%20release%20may%20 2013 (accessed November 2013).
4   Gilmour A, Jones R, Bullock AD. *Dental Foundation Trainers' Expectations of a Dental Graduate.* Final Report. Cardiff: Wales Deanery/Cardiff University; 2012: 1.
5   The NHS (Performers Lists) (England) Regulations 2013, p. 3, ¶30 (1).
6   Ibid.

b) introduce the dental practitioner to all aspects of dental practice in primary care;

c) identify the dental practitioner's personal strengths and weaknesses and balance them through a planned programme of training;

d) promote the oral health of, and quality dental care for, patients;

e) develop and implement peer and self review, and promote awareness of the need for professional education, training and audit as a continuing process; and

f) enable the dental practitioner to—

    (i) make competent and confident professional decisions including decisions for referrals to other services,

    (ii) demonstrate that the dental practitioner is working within the guidelines regarding the ethics and confidentiality of dental practice,

    (iii) implement regulations and guidelines for the delivery of safe practice,

    (iv) know how to obtain appropriate advice on, and practical experience of, legal and financial aspects of practice, and

    (v) demonstrate that the dental practitioner has acquired skill and knowledge in the psychology of care of patients and can work successfully as a member of a practice team.

COPDEND (the UK Committee of Postgraduate Dental Deans and Directors) defines Dental FT as the period of training following initial qualification that builds on the achievements of the dental undergraduate curriculum as defined in *The First Five Years* (General Dental Council) that aims *'to produce a caring competent reflective practitioner able to develop their career in any branch of dentistry to the benefit of patients'*[7] and to demonstrate a level of competence appropriate for independent practice.[8]

While the GDC expects new registrants to be *'well prepared for independent practice'*[9] at the point of registration and therefore *prior* to the commencement of FT, COPDEND[10] have outlined that the demonstration of a level of competence appropriate for independent practice occurs *during* FT. This effectively means that both your Dental School and FT experience doubly ensures that

7   COPDEND. *A Curriculum for UK Dental Foundation Programme Training.* Oxford: COPDEND; 2007. p. 8.

8   COPDEND. *Dental Foundation Training Policy Statement,* ¶2. Available at: www.copdend.org/content. aspx?Group=foundation&Page=foundation_policystatement (accessed November 2013).

9   General Dental Council. *Preparing for Practice: dental team learning outcomes for registration.* London: General Dental Council; 2012. p. 5.

10   COPDEND. *Dental Foundation Training Policy Statement,* ¶2. Available at: www.copdend.org/content. aspx?Group=foundation&Page=foundation_policystatement (accessed November 2013).

you are ready for 'independent practice', which the GDC defines[11] as *'working with autonomy within the GDC Scope of Practice, and own competence, once registered.'* The GDC also goes on to clarify that[12] *'Independent practice does not mean working alone and in isolation, but within the context of the wider dental and healthcare team, and may be under supervision if newly qualified.'*

Although the GDC expects you to be prepared for independent practice COPDEND have recognised that you may need to broaden the scope of practical experience gained at dental school,[13] meaning that you may need to undertake and practise new clinical procedures. Patient safety is of extreme importance and in order to comply with clinical governance requirements, you should not undertake such procedures, for which you have not previously been trained, without direct supervision. You are also not expected at any time to work beyond your level of competence.[14]

RECRUITMENT

'National recruitment' is the centralised process for recruiting FDs into FT across England, Wales and Northern Ireland. It commences with an online application form, of which there were 1318 for 2014, to assess applicants against eligibility criteria. For many applicants FT is the only route available for them to be included on an NHS dental performers list, therefore priority may be given to them over applicants who are exempt from needing to complete FT.[15] Furthermore, some applicants may be considered over others in the recruitment process on the basis of UK immigration legislation. After long-listing has taken place eligible applicants are asked to state a preference order for each of the 78 training schemes via the UK Offers System and invited to attend one of the selection centres across England, Wales and Northern Ireland. For 2014, the selection centre process[16] comprised of a station covering communication in a clinical setting (accounting for 25%) and another

11 General Dental Council. *Preparing for Practice: dental team learning outcomes for registration.* London: General Dental Council; 2012. p. 15.
12 Ibid.
13 COPDEND. *Dental Foundation Training Policy Statement,* ¶23. Available at: www.copdend.org/content. aspx?Group=foundation&Page=foundation_policystatement (accessed November 2013).
14 COPDEND. *Dental Foundation Training Policy Statement,* ¶13. Available at: www.copdend.org/content. aspx?Group=foundation&Page=foundation_policystatement (accessed November 2013).
15 London Shared Services working in partnership with COPDEND for DFT national recruitment 2014. *Nationally Coordinated Dental Foundation Training Recruitment in England, Wales and Northern Ireland 2014 Applicant Guidance, version 1.* London: London Shared Services working in partnership with COPDEND; 2013: 6.
16 Ibid. pp. 10 and 11.

station covering professionalism, management and leadership (accounting for 25%), followed by a Situational Judgement Test (accounting for 50%).

 READING POINT! Patterson F, Ashworth V, Mehra S, *et al.* Could situational judgement tests be used for selection into dental foundation training? *Br Dent J.* 2012: **213**: 23–6.

The scores of all applicants from the selection centres are centrally collated to produce a single national ranking. Successful allocation to a foundation scheme is dependent upon the ranking achieved as a result of selection centre performance with those who score the highest being offered a place on the scheme they most prefer. For 2013, the 968 highest ranked individuals were offered places with 48% of applicants securing their first choice of scheme and 86% one of their top 10 preferred schemes.[17] Offers of a place detailing the Health Education England region and scheme are then made available to successful applicants and once an offer is accepted it cannot be changed to a training placement in another region or scheme. Once all offers have been accepted the list of successful applicants, with their ranking within each scheme, is sent to the region hosting that scheme. Once allocated to a specific scheme the next stage is managed regionally with your ranking potentially being used to inform the allocation process between your training post and a training practice. This is when you generally have the opportunity to meet your potential trainer (Educational Supervisor).

In Scotland, recruitment is administered by NHS Education Scotland and although it starts with an online application process, it involves interviews with trainers during the visitation period. Preferences are then returned to NHS Education Scotland, meaning that applicants rank practices according to preference and trainers rank applicants according to preference. Matching results then indicate the training practice that you are allocated to. A short clearing process may also take place if there are unmatched applicants and vacant training practice posts.

---

17 COPDEND available at: www.copdend.org/content.aspx?Group=press releases&Page=press release dental foundation training places for 2013 announced (accessed November 2013). A second round of applications usually takes place after the last UK dental school finals results have been announced, around June or July, when some successfully matched applicants may be unable to take up their places.

UNDERGRADUATE TO POSTGRADUATE

Perhaps a significant change for the FD is in becoming a 'professional', in that you begin to earn a living from dentistry, as opposed to being an 'amateur' whereby you do not earn a living from dentistry. While working in general dental practice you will be providing dental care to patients in return for either them or the state paying money to the practice, which should in itself highlight the importance of the quality of the care and treatment that you provide. So, another distinction between professionals and amateurs is that the performance of a professional is deemed to be of a higher standard. The way that being a professional differs to being a 'tradesman' is that you are bound by an ethical obligation to act in a certain way in order to uphold the reputation of the profession and to not undermine public confidence in it. This means that you can no longer act as an undergraduate student at, or beyond, the point of GDC registration because you are then automatically considered to become a 'dental professional', meaning that you must act as an ambassador for the profession both inside and outside of the surgery.

The transition from undergraduate student to GDC registrant brings with it a whole host of responsibilities, as outlined in the GDC's *Standards for the Dental Team*,[18] of which you should take note of standard 1.3.2:

> You must make sure you do not bring the profession into disrepute.

However your internal ethical compass is set, it should be pointed to align to the GDC's expectations, thereby helping you to visualise the boundary lines that you should not cross as a dental professional. The expectation for you to observe and conform to the standards set out by the GDC is also reinforced in clause 17.7 of the Foundation Contract.

> *If it is not right, do not do it: If it is not true, do not do it.*
>
> —Marcus Aurelius Antoninus (121–180 AD)

NOVICE TO ADVANCED BEGINNER

As a new registrant, at the starting point of your FT journey, you are deemed to be a *safe beginner*,[19] with the Dreyfus model of skill acquisition[20] asserting

---

18 General Dental Council. *Standards for the Dental Team*. London: General Dental Council; 2013.
19 General Dental Council. *Preparing for Practice: dental team learning outcomes for registration*. London: General Dental Council; 2012. p. 6.
20 Dreyfus HL, Dreyfus SE. *Mind Over Machine: the power of human intuition and expertise in the age of the computer*. Oxford: Basil Blackwell; 1986.

that this journey arguably ends at the *advanced beginner* stage. This model can be used to describe your progress throughout the year in the development of skills or competencies and defines an acceptable level for the assessment of competence or capability. Based on the work of Dreyfus and Dreyfus[21] we can depict different skill levels as a ladder that you walk up throughout your career (*see* Table 1.1), with each rung representing a different level with discrete characteristics.

TABLE 1.1 Dental skill acquisition

Ladder rung	Stage	Standard of work	Characteristics
6	Expert	Excellence achieved with relative ease	Deep tacit understanding across area of practice, able to take responsibility for going beyond existing standards and creating own interpretations
5	Proficient	Fully acceptable standard achieved routinely	Sees overall 'picture', decision-making more confident and deals with complex situations holistically
4	Competent	Fit for purpose, although may lack refinement	Copes with complex situations through deliberate analysis and is able to achieve most tasks using own judgement
3	Advanced beginner	Procedures more likely to be completed to an acceptable standard	Working knowledge of key aspects of practice; exit point of FT
2	Safe beginner	Procedures likely to be completed to an acceptable standard	Working knowledge of key aspects of practice but supervision required for execution; entry point of FT
1	Novice	Unlikely to be satisfactory unless closely supervised	'Textbook' knowledge with limited application to practice; requires instruction

So, FT helps you to climb from the *safe beginner* rung upwards to the advanced beginner rung, helping to guide your own journey up the remaining rungs throughout your professional career.

Contrary to popular belief, a 1990 study[22] by Ericsson found that it is not always talent or innate genius that makes you an expert but rather the hours

---

21 Adapted from The Institute of Conservation. *Professional Standards for Conservation.* London: Institute of Conservation; 2003. Available at: www.sld.demon.co.uk/dreyfus.pdf (accessed November 2013).

22 Ericsson KA, Krampe R Th, Tesch-Romer C. The role of deliberate practice in the acquisition of expert performance. *Psychol Rev.* 1993; **100**: 393–4.

that you are willing to put in. In his book, Malcolm Gladwell[23] references this study asserting that the key to truly mastering a skill is, to a large extent, a matter of deliberately practising that skill for a total of around 10 000 hours. This has been calculated on the basis of performing that skill 20 hours a week, for 50 weeks a year, for 10 years. Using a comparative calculation, if you were to deliberately practice over the same hours worked as in FT for the foreseeable future (taking the same amount of holidays), this would calculate to over 6 years before you could be considered an expert.

DELIBERATE PRACTICE

This is not just a matter of practising your skills on phantom heads for over 6 years. It involves:
- evaluating and assessing your success
- monitoring your performance through reflection, and
- improving aspects of your performance that you are not so good at.

TERMINOLOGY FOR STARTERS

TABLE 1.2 Foundation Training terminology

Name	Previous or related name	General role
Foundation Training (FT)	DF1 or Vocational Training	A one year period of training following initial qualification that builds on the achievements of the dental undergraduate curriculum. It aims* 'to produce a caring competent reflective practitioner able to develop their career'
Local education and training board (LETB) hosted by Health Education England (HEE)	Postgraduate deanery	They bring education, training and development together locally, to improve the quality of care and treatment of patients through the development of skills and values for the workforce
COPDEND (UK Committee of Postgraduate Dental Deans and Directors)	–	Governs and leads UK FT
Director of Postgraduate Dental Education	Postgraduate dental dean	Commissions and manages the delivery of postgraduate dental education and training in a region

---

23 Gladwell M. *Outliers: the story of success.* 1st ed. New York: Little, Brown and Company; 2008.

Name	Previous or related name	General role
Associate director of Foundation Training	Associate dean for Foundation Training	Oversees and strategically manages the commissioning and delivery of FT in a region
FTPD (Foundation Training programme director)	Vocational Training Adviser	Commissions and manages the delivery of the competencies within the COPDEND Dental Foundation Training Curriculum to a cohort of Foundation Dentists (FDs) in a scheme. They also recruit and support Educational Supervisors and FDs
ES (educational supervisor)	Vocational (in practice[†]) Trainer	Responsible for overseeing the educational progress and day-to-day clinical supervision of the FD. The ES may also be the FD's employer
FD (Foundation Dentist)	Vocational Dental Practitioner	New registrant who has successfully been allocated an ES. Their skills learned as an undergraduate are built upon during FT

* COPDEND. *A Curriculum for UK Dental Foundation Programme Training.* Oxford: COPDEND; 2007. p. 8.
† COPDEND. *Guidance notes on the Foundation Contract.* Revised. Oxford: COPDEND; 2013.

So, your position is as an FD working under the supervision of an ES in a training practice, after being allocated to an FT scheme accountable to one or more LETBs on behalf of HEE.

The FTPD manages both the ES and the FD, which some LETBs have identified as a conflict of interest. Although this has traditionally been managed well by FTPDs since the inception of Vocational Training, there is an increasing approach for the responsibility to support the FD and to manage the ES to be separated. This involves an *FD Support Tutor*, whose responsibility is to support FDs working towards and achieving FT goals and an Associate Dean's responsibility to quality manage and develop your ES, as well as commissioning the study day programme. For you, this has the effect of depending upon one individual for arranging your study day programme and another to provide you with support as well as acting as the 'honest broker' between you and your ES.

POSTGRADUATE DENTAL EDUCATION

Postgraduate dental education encompasses:
- Foundation Training
- Dental Core Training
- Dentists with Enhanced Skills Training (Dentists with Special Interests)

- Specialty Training (as a specialty registrar)
- Competency Assessment
- Remedial training for registrants in difficulty
- Short courses for dental professionals, including core continuing professional development (CPD)
- Section 63 courses for dentists within the general dental services and salaried dental services
- Pre-registration training for dental care professionals, and
- Additional skills training for dental professionals (as specified in the *GDC Scope of Practice*[24])

The commissioning of education for short courses and Section 63 courses is currently performed locally by Postgraduate Dental Tutors and approved by the Postgraduate Dental Dean. Given that postgraduate dental education is considered as the continuous progression of FT, momentum is building for FT and other postgraduate dental education to be commissioned by the same individual (a Patch Associate Dean) in a designated locality on behalf of that specific LETB. Through engagement with various stakeholders (such as the NHS England Area Team and Public Health England) the individual would supposedly have a better insight into what the local dental workforce's needs are across a patch, resulting in more effective commissioning of postgraduate dental education for that workforce. This approach would amalgamate the traditional roles of the FTPD and the Postgraduate Dental Tutor.

STARTING REQUIREMENTS

- FDs are appointed by a national recruitment process and allocated a ranking, enabling allocation to a training practice within a training scheme or patch. So, it is important to have received a confirmed place on a training scheme or patch.
- You will need to have been registered with the GDC as a dentist, which can only be achieved once you have completed a recognised degree (such as a Bachelor of Dental Surgery).
- You will be required to agree to and sign the nationally agreed Foundation Contract and a LETB specific Educational Agreement.
- In England, as you will work as a performer in the NHS you will need to apply to be included on the NHS England national dental performers

---

24 General Dental Council. *Scope of Practice*. London: General Dental Council; 2013.

list, a process which will also require clearance of a Disclosure and Barring Service check (formerly a Criminal Records Bureau check). Although the NHS (Performers Lists) (England) Regulations 2013 outline that you can perform primary dental services despite not being included on the national dental performers list during the first 3 months of Foundation Training,[25] this 'period of grace' is generally for those experiencing unavoidable delays in the application process. It is important to be included on the national dental performers list from the outset.

- As you will be an employee of the practice (i.e. of the ES or the practice owner) you will need to have the legal right to work in the UK for a period of a year working 35 hours a week.
- For salary administration purposes you will need to provide your P45 to your ES or practice owner, or, failing that, the information requested of you within a 'Starter Checklist'.[26]

THE FOUNDATION CONTRACT

The Foundation Contract is the contract of employment that your Foundation Trainer will ask you to read, understand, encourage you to ask questions about and then ultimately agree to by signing. It has been approved as the national standard by COPDEND and underpins your FT experience. The contract has been written in the context of three main parties: (1) the FD, (2) the ES and (3) the practice owner. Often the ES and the practice owner will be the same person. Throughout this book we will refer to the various clauses within the Foundation Contract.

EDUCATIONAL AGREEMENT

The Educational Agreement is not a contract of employment. Its purpose is rather to set out the terms of your participation on the LETB training scheme that you have been allocated to; hence the agreement may differ regionally. Usual terms of participation are that you are expected to work under the direction of the ES and that you complete the various requirements of the programme such as attending the study day programme and weekly tutorials in practice.

---

25   The NHS (Performers Lists) (England) Regulations 2013, ¶31 (2).
26   HM Revenue & Customs. Available at: www.hmrc.gov.uk/working/forms/paye-forms.htm (accessed November 2013).

COMPLETION

The satisfactory completion of the Foundation Training programme is decided by the Postgraduate Dental Dean or Director who awards you a certificate of completion of training at the end of the year upon successfully demonstrating the competencies outlined in the COPDEND Dental Foundation Training Curriculum (*see* Chapter 4). There is a complex relationship between outcomes, performance and experience which is time dependent.[27]

In England the certificate of completion needs to be sent to NHS England[28] who will then alter your status on the national dental performers list from 'trainee' to 'dental performer'. You will also be issued with a Vocational Training number from the NHS Business Services Authority (BSA).

The criteria for satisfactory completion is broadly the same for all FDs, as per the nationally agreed Foundation Contract; however, there may be regional differences as per the Educational Agreement. Table 1.3 provides a broad outline of the criteria.

TABLE 1.3 Criteria for satisfactory completion

Requirement	How monitored/assessed
Completion of the study day programme (usually a minimum of 30 study days*)	The *Reflection on study days* section in e-PDP (Electronic Personal Development Plan), validated by your FTPD
Completion of a full training year (1 year of full-time employment)	Feedback from your ES, together with the *Clinical Experience Log* section in e-PDP
Attendance of weekly tutorials with your ES in practice	The *Tutorial Reflection* section in e-PDP, validated by your ES
Satisfactory clinical experience	Regularly updating the *Clinical Experience Log* section in e-PDP
Completion of an FT portfolio of evidence (*see* Chapter 9)	Assessed by your FTPD or an ES in your scheme
Completion of the required number of assessments	Completing the *Early Stage Peer Reviews (ESPRs)*, *Dental Evaluation of Performance Tools (A'DEP'Ts)*, *Dental Case-Based Discussions (D-CbDs)* and *Patient Assessment Questionnaire (PAQ)* on e-PDP together with your ES
Presentation of a case report[†]	Presentation to a group usually consisting of the FDs and ESs from the scheme along with the FTPD

---

27   COPDEND. Dental Foundation Training Policy Statement, ¶5. Available at: www.copdend.org/content.aspx?Group=foundation&Page=foundation_policystatement (accessed November 2013).

28   The NHS (Performers Lists) (England) Regulations 2013, ¶33 3(a)(iii).

Requirement	How monitored/assessed
Clinical audit[‡]	Completing the *Audit* section in e-PDP
Completion of the e-PDP	Timely and satisfactory completion of the various areas outlined in e-PDP, including reflections

[*] COPDEND. Dental Foundation Training Policy Statement, ¶19. Available at: www.copdend.org/content.aspx?Group=foundation&Page=foundation_policystatement (accessed November 2013).

[†] COPDEND. Dental Foundation Training Policy Statement, ¶18. Available at: www.copdend.org/content.aspx?Group=foundation&Page=foundation_policystatement (accessed November 2013).

[‡] Ibid.

COPDEND have expressed a wish to move towards a system of satisfactory completion of Dental Foundation Training[29] by *'introducing a formal robust assessment framework comprising a series of formative assessments which combine to deliver a summative assessment at the end of the foundation training period'* but this is not active at the time of writing.

CLINICAL EXPERIENCE

Every FD is allocated a notional activity level of 1875 UDAs (Units of Dental Activity) by NHS England to complete within the FT year. However, this is *not* a target, since there is no financial adjustment levied by NHS England for under- or over-performance, and it is not a true indication of your clinical progress for two reasons. First, UDAs do not measure the range of clinical procedures performed, and, second, UDAs do not measure any private treatment that you may need to perform during FT for cosmetic purposes. Therefore, it is more likely that your FTPD will use e-PDP to monitor the breadth and depth of your clinical experience by virtue of whether you:

- have performed most of the procedures listed in the Clinical Experience Log section of e-PDP, and
- appear as an outlier for the amount of procedures performed against your peers.

The NHS national care pathways advocate three levels of clinicians, with Level 1 clinicians relating to general dental practitioners (GDPs) working at a level consistent with the completion of FT. This national approach clearly emphasises the importance of you being able to demonstrate adequate clinical experience by the end of the year, which could result in clinical treatment

---

29 COPDEND. *Dental Foundation Training Policy Statement,* ¶29. Available at: www.copdend.org/content.aspx?Group=foundation&Page=foundation_policystatement (accessed November 2013).

procedure targets being introduced. However, as each training practice serves different communities with discrete treatment needs, you may sometimes not be able to perform certain procedures as often as you would like on account of there being little clinical need. Instead of completing the year without experiencing these clinical procedures there could be provision for you to experience these procedures in a different clinical environment.

Table 1.4 outlines the range of clinical procedures that you should be performing and recording in your *Clinical Experience Log* section of e-PDP during the year.

TABLE 1.4 Expected range of clinical procedures

Purpose of treatment	Clinical procedure
Patient examination and diagnosis	Examinations
	Radiographs
	Impressions
Treatment planning and patient management	Treatment and planning
	Children (routine)
	Children in pain
	Adults in pain
Health promotion/disease prevention	Health promotion
	Preventive education plan
	Fluoride varnish
Medical and dental emergencies	Basic life support (BLS)/medical emergencies training
	Medical emergencies
	Dental trauma
Anaesthesia, pain and anxiety control	Local anaesthetic
	Anxious patients
Periodontal therapy and management of soft tissue	Six-point periodontal chart
	Simple scale
	Root surface debridement (RSD)
Hard and soft tissue surgery	Extraction erupted teeth
	Extraction buried roots
	Simple surgical procedures
	Surgery involving flap, sutures

Purpose of treatment	Clinical procedure
Non-surgical management	Prescribing
	Referrals
	Denture alterations
Restoration of teeth	Rubber dam
	Amalgam restorations
	Anterior composite restorations
	Posterior composite restorations
	Root canal treatment incisor/canine
	Root canal treatment premolar
	Root canal treatment molar
	Crowns/veneers
	Bridge – resin retained
	Bridge – conventional
	Fissure sealant
	Glass ionomer cement (GIC)
Replacement of teeth	Posts including amalgam cores
	Acrylic complete
	Acrylic partial
	Cobalt-chromium partial

NON-COMPLETION

Ideally all FDs will complete their FT; however, there are times when this is unfortunately not the case. Examples of such times are as follows.

- When you have had an extended period of absence from your training. Although measures are usually taken by LETBs to provide you with additional clinical experience at your training practice or within another practice, to help ensure that your training has been of 1-year duration, there is no compulsion to do so. If for any reason your training period has to be extended to enable satisfactory completion of the programme, you will be asked to enter into a new contract.
- If you are dismissed from your scheme by failing to attend (or failing to make up any missed) study days, consistently failing to maintain e-PDP or displaying unprofessional conduct by contravening legal or regulatory guidelines.
- Failing to comply with your ES, FTPD or Dean's reasonable requests.

- Serious concerns raised regarding your competency in any of the four domains outlined in the COPDEND Dental Foundation Training Curriculum (*see* Chapter 4) that cannot be remediated.
- An irrevocable breakdown in your relationship with your ES leading to your ES providing notice of termination of your employment.
- If you resign from your training practice without consulting your FTPD, Associate Director of Foundation Training or Director of Postgraduate Dental Education.

NHS England is ultimately responsible for deciding whether dentists who have not completed FT (and are not exempt from this requirement) have the skills and experience for admission onto the national dental performers list on the advice of the Postgraduate Dental Dean.

EXPECTATIONS

COPDEND have outlined the following expectations of the FD[30] in the general dental services:

- enter into a nationally agreed contract of employment (the Foundation Contract)
- attend the practice/clinic for the agreed hours and perform such clinical duties as appropriate for patient care and personal learning needs
- determine, record and address personal learning needs with the support of his or her ES(s) and supervisors and the Dental Foundation Training e-PDP (assessments and reflection)
- maintain an up-to-date e-Portfolio, including timely completion of the educational activities described therein, and discuss the outcomes regularly with his or her ES/FTPD
- take an active part in weekly tutorials and study days and other educational activities
- to be assessed once each month throughout FT (except for Month 1) using A'DEP'T.
- to be assessed once each month throughout FT using the D-CbD tool
- to be assessed once using a PAQ
- to complete the Clinical Experience Log, Assessment Log, CPD and

---

30 COPDEND. *Dental Foundation Training Portfolio & Assessment: user guide*, ¶9. Available at: www.copdend.org/data/files/Foundation/Dental%20Foundation%20Training%20Portfolio%20User%20Guide%5B1%5D.pdf (accessed November 2013).

Education Log and Personal Development Plan regularly each month as appropriate, and share this information with his or her ES and FTPD

- reflect on his or her own practice throughout the training, including the completion of a written reflection form for his or her e-Portfolio at least once each month (or weekly during the first 8 weeks of FT).

COPDEND have also outlined the following expectations of the ES[31] in the general dental services:

- employ his or her FD as a salaried assistant under the terms of the contract and, before he or she starts work, deposit a copy of the signed contract with the Postgraduate Dental Dean or Director
- work in the same premises as the FD, in a surgery to which he or she has good access for no fewer than 3 days per week
- provide the FD with adequate administrative support and the full-time assistance of a suitably experienced dental nurse
- provide satisfactory facilities (including an adequate supply of handpieces and instruments, sufficient to allow them to be sterilised between patients) and relevant opportunities so that a wide range of NHS practice is experienced, and so far as is reasonably possible the FD is fully occupied
- conduct an initial assessment interview, and complete informal ESPR assessment during the first 4 weeks of Dental Foundation Training, to identify strengths and weaknesses and identify training priorities and learning objectives
- be available for guidance in both clinical and administrative matters: provide help on request or where necessary
- assess and monitor the FD's progress and professional development using the e-Portfolio, including the completion of assessments and monitoring forms, and provision of feedback as required
- provide feedback to the FTPD as required
- prepare and conduct hourly tutorials on a weekly basis (within normal practice hours), some of which will be used for assessment and feedback to the FD
- acquire the skills necessary to undertake the role of ES, including skills as assessor

---

31   COPDEND. *Dental Foundation Training Portfolio & Assessment: user guide*, pp. 9 and 10. Available at: www.copdend.org/data/files/Foundation/Dental%20Foundation%20Training%20Portfolio%20 User%20Guide%5B1%5D.pdf (accessed November 2013).

- attend trainer meetings, study days and/or scheme assessment sessions as per contract
- provide reference material for the use of the FD.

In the hospital and salaried dental services there is an expectation for FDs to be assessed once using a Multi-Source Feedback tool, either mini-PAT (peer assessment tool) or TAB (team assessment of behaviours). This may also prove beneficial to FDs in the general dental services, as the modern general dental practice involves working with a multidisciplinary team.

YOUR ES

Your ES, otherwise known as the in practice trainer, is not simply an educational supervisor but also a clinical supervisor.[32] Your ES is your mentor throughout the year responsible for day-to-day clinical supervision, facilitating and carrying out assessments and ensuring appropriate workload.[33] As with other trades and crafts since time immemorial, you and your ES must make a pact at the beginning of the year, outlining your respective roles and responsibilities, which is documented in the Educational Agreement section of e-PDP. The relationship you have with your ES must therefore be open, honest and trusting. You should not be afraid to work with your ES to help shine a light on your hidden weaknesses, as this will help you to strengthen them. The role of the ES includes teaching and assessing your demonstration of the competencies within all four domains outlined in the COPDEND Dental Foundation Training Curriculum.

YOUR FTPD

The role of your FTPD includes commissioning a study day programme with the aim of covering the competencies outlined in the COPDEND Dental Foundation Training Curriculum. Your FTPD also ensures that you encounter the best-possible training environment and practice experience by being involved in the selection, development[34] and performance management of your ES. More importantly for you, however, is that your FTPD is there to

32 COPDEND. *Dental Foundation Training Policy Statement,* ¶35. Available at: www.copdend.org/content.aspx?Group=foundation&Page=foundation_policystatement (accessed November 2013).

33 COPDEND. *Dental Foundation Training Policy Statement,* ¶34. Available at: www.copdend.org/content.aspx?Group=foundation&Page=foundation_policystatement (accessed November 2013).

34 COPDEND. *Dental Foundation Training Policy Statement,* ¶30. Available at: www.copdend.org/content.aspx?Group=foundation&Page=foundation_policystatement (accessed November 2013).

provide you with pastoral support and to provide you with a helping hand in overcoming any difficulties that your ES is unable to assist you with throughout the year. The FTPD has regular contact with your ES, such as at trainers' meetings, and therefore is able to feed back to them regarding your experience, unless the matter you discuss is of a confidential or personal nature. Some regions will invite you to complete a confidential review form about your FT practice, experience and progress at regular intervals throughout the year, which is not disclosed to your trainer. The Postgraduate Dental Director's decision to permit you to complete the FT programme is informed by your FTPD.

General dental practice

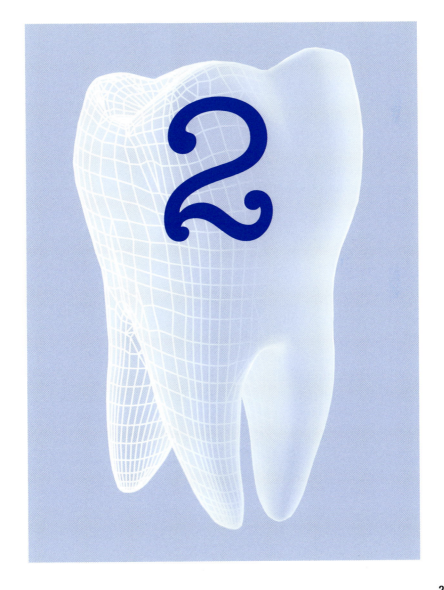

Ninety-five per cent of oral healthcare in the UK is provided in primary care, mostly in general dental practice.[35] For the general public, GDPs are usually the first point of contact, connecting them if necessary to other healthcare services. Although the majority of FT posts consist of placements in general dental practice there are also a number within the salaried dental services. As an FD working in general dental practice you will be expected to see the full range of patients, offering the full range of NHS dental treatment and even some non-NHS treatment.

Unlike at dental school, during FT you will tend to see the same patients after completing their treatments, which enables you to follow your work through and see first hand your successes and failures. This is great, as you will get to know what works and what doesn't.

SUPERVISION

In dental school it is likely that your clinical skills were taught in a protected environment, with consultants helping you to plan treatment and clinical instructors peering over your shoulder to supervise your clinical work. In FT, the environment is less protected in that you will be less supervised than before, but, nevertheless, training practices operate an 'open door' policy whereby you are welcome to interrupt your ES or an associate to gain assistance.

'Supervision' in FT refers to a focused dialogue, with a supervisor, about your work and is aimed at developing your professional practice and improving patient care. These conversations must be open and honest and can take place either informally when popping into your colleague's room through his or her open door or formally within in-practice tutorials. The word 'super' in supervision implies the action of helping to stretch or improve your skills, while the word 'vision' implies doing this through observation. The two domains of supervision defined by Launer[36] are:

1. *performance* – this refers to your clinical progress being overseen
2. *development* – this refers to your personal, professional and educational development over time.

35 Faculty of General Dental Practice (UK). Available at: www.fgdp.org.uk/research.ashx (accessed July 2013).
36 Launer J. *Supervision, Mentoring and Coaching: one-to-one learning encounter in medical education.* Edinburgh: Association for the Study of Medical Education; 2006.

ACTION POINT! It can be difficult asking for assistance from your ES when you have a patient in the chair, mid procedure. Agree a code with your dental nurse which, when stated, indicates a desire for him or her to call your ES into your surgery.

MATERIALS AND EQUIPMENT

Considering your undergraduate experience in a large, multispecialty hospital environment, it should come as no surprise that the resources available to you in general practice may be a little more limited. However, as the standard of care in both environments should be the same, it is unlikely that you will need to ask your ES to purchase any further equipment or materials than is already available. However, if you do feel that patients could benefit from a particular piece of equipment or material, don't be afraid to ask your ES or the practice owner but do remember to be realistic. If you have concerns about the equipment or materials available in practice, do approach your ES in the first instance or otherwise you can raise this with your FTPD.

It is also important that you understand how to maintain the equipment that you shall be routinely using during the year, such as the dental chair and suction unit. In fact an understanding of the considerations to be made during the selection, care and maintenance of equipment is a COPDEND curriculum competency[37] that you are expected to demonstrate during FT.

THE NHS LANDSCAPE

The *Health and Social Care Act 2012* formed the basis of an extensive reorganisation of the structure of the NHS in England in 2013, with the changes aiming to empower patients and local clinicians to jointly make decisions about local NHS services. The current NHS landscape can be simplified into: (1) NHS service delivery, (2) monitoring the NHS and (3) the NHS workforce.

---

37 Committee of Postgraduate Dental Deans and Directors UK (COPDEND). *Interim Dental Foundation Training Curriculum & Assessment Framework Guidance 2013–2014.* Oxford: COPDEND; 2013. Management & leadership domain, ¶1 (5).

NHS service delivery

TABLE 2.1 Bodies involved with NHS service delivery

Body	Function
Department of Health	Supports the Secretary of State for Health, setting national policy and legislation
NHS England	Independent body managing the NHS budget and commissioning services including all dental services Local professional networks for dentistry work with each area team of NHS England
Clinical commissioning groups	Groups of general practitioners responsible for commissioning non-dental local health services
Health and wellbeing boards	Forums where key leaders from the health and care system work together to improve the health and wellbeing of their local population and reduce health inequalities

Monitoring the NHS

TABLE 2.2 Bodies involved with monitoring

Body	Function
Care Quality Commission (CQC)	To ensure that care provided meets national standards of quality and safety. The CQC is considered to be the independent regulator of all health and social care services in England
Monitor	Promotes the provision of healthcare services that are effective, efficient and economic, and maintains or improves the quality of services
Healthwatch England	To ensure that the voices of patients and those who use services reach the ears of the decision-makers. Healthwatch England is considered to be the independent consumer champion for health and social care in England

The NHS workforce

TABLE 2.3 Bodies involved with the NHS workforce

Body	Function
Health Education England	Responsible for the education, training and personal development of every member of NHS staff, and recruiting for values
LETB	Develops, educates and trains the current and future NHS workforce
The National Institute for Health and Care Excellence (NICE)	Produces guidance, quality standards and other products to support health, public health and social care practitioners in providing the best possible quality care and the best value for money
NHS Employers	To provide expertise in human resources. NHS Employers is considered as the voice of employers in the NHS
NHS Leadership Academy	Develops outstanding leadership in health, in order to improve people's health and their experience of the NHS

NHS DENTISTRY

Operationally, a dental provider has a fixed contract with NHS England that determines the amount of NHS activity expected to be performed in return for an annual payment paid to the dental provider in 12 monthly instalments. UDAs are the currency used to monitor quantitative performance of NHS activity, and providers can deliver their contract through engaging dental performers. As an FD you are a dental performer working under the NHS (General Dental Services Contracts) Regulations 2005, but your NHS activity is separate to the contracted NHS activity of the training practice that you work within.

The General Dental Services Contract[38] lays down a requirement to provide *'all proper and necessary dental care and treatment'*[39] to meet the reasonable needs of patients that patients are willing to undergo.[40] Furthermore, the contract outlines a requirement *'to secure the oral health of the patient'*.[41] As asserted by the World Health Organization, oral health means more than simply having 'good teeth', it allows us to speak, smile, kiss, touch, taste, chew, swallow and cry.

38 The Standard General Dental Services Contract, revised April 2013. Available at: www.gov.uk/govern ment/publications/standard-general-dental-services-contract-and-personal-dental-services-agreement (accessed November 2013).
39 The Standard General Dental Services Contract, Clause 74.
40 The Standard General Dental Services Contract, Clause 74.1.
41 The Standard General Dental Services Contract, Clause 47.5.

As you shall be working in the NHS general dental services there is an expectation that you shall provide mandatory services to patients, which includes urgent treatment and the following:

- examination
- diagnosis
- advice and planning of treatment
- preventive care and treatment
- periodontal treatment
- conservative treatment
- surgical treatment
- supply and repair of dental appliances
- the taking of radiographs
- the supply of listed drugs and listed appliances
- the issue of prescriptions.[42]

From the General Dental Services Contract (and the Personal Dental Services Agreement) we can infer that all treatments are technically available to patients under the NHS and subsequently there cannot be a practice policy of specific treatments only being available on a private basis if they are clinically necessary to secure a patient's oral health. Understanding which items of treatment fall within the NHS regulations, and being able to discuss the consequences of this with the patient in a manner that they can understand, is a COPDEND curriculum competency[43] that you are expected to demonstrate during FT.

NHS care and treatment is best described in terms of courses of treatment as opposed to UDAs. A course of treatment[44] comprises:

- an examination of a patient and assessment of their oral health;
- the planning of any treatment to be provided to that patient as a result of that examination and assessment; and
- the provision of any planned treatment (including any treatment planned at a time other than the time of the initial examination) to that patient.

 ACTION POINT! Ask your ES whether the training practice has a policy for providing specific treatments under the NHS and privately.

---

42   The Standard General Dental Services Contract, Clause 76.

43   Committee of Postgraduate Dental Deans and Directors UK (COPDEND). *Interim Dental Foundation Training Curriculum & Assessment Framework Guidance 2013–2014*. Oxford: COPDEND; 2013 communication domain, ¶2 (6).

44   The NHS (General Dental Services Contracts) Regulations 2005, p. 1, ¶2 (1).

THINKING POINT! If an item of treatment, such as a posterior composite, is not appropriate on the NHS on the basis of it not being clinically justified, would it be ethical for it to be available privately?

Six-monthly dental check-ups have been customary in the General Dental Service, but the NICE clinical guidelines *Dental Recall: Recall Interval between Routine Dental Examinations*[45] has directed a move towards making NHS dental services in England and Wales more oriented to prevention and more clinically effective in meeting patients' needs. The guidance recommends that the time interval between oral health reviews should be tailored to each patient based on an assessment of disease levels and risk from oral disease. This has led to the now common practice of using a red, amber or green classification to risk-assess individual patients for developing oral disease including caries, periodontal disease and oral cancer. The precise criteria used to justify specific risk classification is not based on a mathematical formula but rather a clinical judgement.

The stepwise approach to providing dentistry that you would have learned at undergraduate level also applies within the general dental services, whereby the stabilisation of oral disease precludes the provision of definitive treatment. The 'treatment lock' model advocated by the Department of Health describes how patients at higher risk of dental disease (such as the red category) should be prevented from accessing more advanced care, such as the laboratory fabricated items available within NHS Band 3, until they are able to demonstrate entering a lower-risk level (such as the green category).

 THINKING POINT! Regardless of the 'treatment lock' model, many FDs are concerned that not providing all operative treatment that a patient requires within the same course of treatment could constitute 'supervised neglect' even in the presence of good clinical records. Could supervised neglect be deemed as:
- the advanced restoration of carious cavities without first reviewing patient compliance with advice aimed at preventing caries and without the demonstration of caries stabilisation, or
- the review of successful compliance with caries prevention advice along with the demonstration of caries stabilisation, prior to advanced restoration?

---

45   NICE Clinical Guideline 19. *Dental Recall: recall interval between routine dental examinations.* October 2004.

FP17 forms act as the 'claims' for NHS activity performed that are submitted to the NHS BSA for processing. It is imperative that these forms are completed accurately for work performed by you bearing your unique performer number, as it is considered inappropriate for FP17 forms to be submitted for work performed by yourself but bearing a non-FD performer's number. Often, however, more than one performer performs an NHS course of treatment; for example, when your ES or another performer in the practice assists you with performing treatment. The general view in these circumstances is that the FP17 claim form submission should bear the performer number of whichever performer performed the majority of the treatment.

The National Health Service (Dental Charges) Regulations 2005 and the scope of dentistry provided within National Health Service (General Dental Services Contracts) Regulations 2005 fall outwith the remit of this book; however, your ES will provide you with guidance on this, supplemented by your scheme's study day programme.

 READING POINT! You can access the following regulations at:
- The National Health Service (General Dental Services Contracts) Regulations 2005: www.legislation.gov.uk/uksi/2005/3361/regulation/2/made
- The National Health Service (Dental Charges) Regulations 2005: www.legislation.gov.uk/uksi/2005/3477/schedules/made

DELIVERING BETTER ORAL HEALTH

Delivering Better Oral Health: An Evidence-Based Toolkit for Prevention[46] provides guidance to all the members of the dental team on evidence-based prevention, but its messages can also be used for disease stabilisation. After first outlining the levels of evidence to be used throughout, the guidance outlines the following eight sections covering discrete areas in which to prevent and control oral diseases.

1. Principles of toothbrushing for oral health
2. Increasing fluoride availability
3. Healthy eating advice
4. Identifying sugar-free medicines

---

46 Department of Health. *Delivering Better Oral Health: an evidence-based toolkit for prevention.* 2nd ed. London: the Department of Health and the British Association for the Study of Community Dentistry; 2009. 3rd edition not published at time of writing.

5. Improving periodontal health
6. Stop smoking guidance
7. Accessing alcohol misuse support
8. Prevention of erosion

The evidence-based messages highlighted for each area in this list should not be delivered through the giving of advice to patients relying on a 'dentist knows best' relationship but rather as part of an open dialogue helping to activate a behaviour change. Although it is recognised that you will be unable to directly motivate a patient to change his or her lifestyle behaviour, the patient can activate his or her readiness to change.[47] Providing appropriate, relevant and up to date preventive education to individual patients in a manner that inspires motivation for change is a COPDEND curriculum competency[48] that you are expected to demonstrate during FT.

Although *Delivering Better Oral Health* advocates twice-yearly[49] fluoride varnish applications for children aged between 3 and 18 years, this may be seen to contravene the National Health Service (Dental Charges) Regulations 2005 if those appointments are for urgent treatment. This is because schedule 4, regulation 4(5) for Urgent treatment under Band 1 charge does not include 'surface application as primary preventive measures of sealants and topical fluoride preparations'.[50] However, the consensus view is that even if you see a child or adolescent for urgent care, you can apply fluoride varnish, as this may be the only opportunity that you have of seeing the patient to reduce their caries experience.

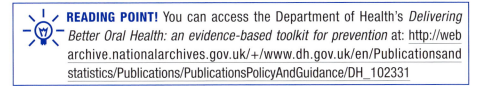

READING POINT! You can access the Department of Health's *Delivering Better Oral Health: an evidence-based toolkit for prevention* at: http://web archive.nationalarchives.gov.uk/+/www.dh.gov.uk/en/Publicationsand statistics/Publications/PublicationsPolicyAndGuidance/DH_102331

The modern general dental practice team is multidisciplinary, comprising

47   Rollnick S, Kinnersley P, Stott N. Methods of helping patients with behaviour change. *BMJ*. 1993; **307**(6897): 188–90.
48   Committee of Postgraduate Dental Deans and Directors UK (COPDEND). *Interim Dental Foundation Training Curriculum & Assessment Framework Guidance 2013–2014*. Oxford: COPDEND; 2013 communication domain, ¶1 (9).
49   Department of Health. *Delivering Better Oral Health: an evidence-based toolkit for prevention*. 2nd ed. London: the Department of Health and the British Association for the Study of Community Dentistry; 2009. p. 21.
50   The National Health Service (Dental Charges) Regulations 2005 S1 R4(1).

team members with wide-ranging roles as shown in Table 2.4. The roles of clinical team members are clearly outlined in the GDC's *Scope of Practice.*[51]

TABLE 2.4 Roles of the general dental practice team

Team Member	Description
Provider	Holds a contract (General Dental Services or Personal Dental Services) with NHS England and has the responsibility for that entire contract. They are normally the practice owner and are often, but not necessarily, NHS dental performers
Associate/ performer	Registered dentist and NHS dental performer who is contractually engaged by a provider to work under their contract. They are usually, but not necessarily, self-employed and although not in contract with NHS England they are responsible for working within the NHS regulations.
Dental nurse	Registered dental professional who provides clinical and other support to registrants and patients.* The dental nurse must be either GDC registered or enrolled and waiting to start on a recognised programme that will lead to GDC registration
Dental nurse with additional skills	Registered dental nurse who, with further training and assessment, could develop a range of further skills including the ability to apply fluoride varnish either on prescription from a dentist or direct as part of a structured dental health programme. Dental nurses do not diagnose disease or treatment plan†
Dental hygienist	Registered dental professional who helps patients to maintain their oral health by preventing and treating periodontal disease and promoting good oral health practice. They can carry out their full scope of practice without prescription and without the patient having to see a dentist first‡
Dental therapist	Registered dental professional who carries out certain items of dental treatment direct to patients or under prescription from a dentist. They are increasingly being employed to perform NHS dentistry in dental practices dependent upon local arrangements
Receptionist	Non-clinical role acting as the point of patient contact for administrative purposes such as managing appointments, taking payments and answering queries
Practice manager	Non-clinical role involving the day-to-day running of the practice and duties such as ordering materials, arranging equipment repair and managing staff payroll. A practice manager may also be the service's CQC registered manager, who is in charge of regulated activities

* General Dental Council. *Scope of Practice.* London: General Dental Council; 2013. p. 4.

† General Dental Council. *Scope of Practice.* London: General Dental Council; 2013. p. 5.

‡ General Dental Council. *Direct Access Guidance.* London: General Dental Council; 2013.

---

51 General Dental Council. *Scope of Practice*. London: General Dental Council; 2013.

Despite being employed, and being somewhat led by your dental nurse and practice manager, you must remember that as a registered dentist the GDC holds you primarily responsible for ensuring that all standards relevant to patient care are met in your surgery room. In fact the GDC would potentially hold you accountable for all standards relevant to patient care in the entire practice if you were the only dentist working at the time.

TIME MANAGEMENT

Time management can be challenging for the FD, with a 2012 survey conducted by Cardiff University revealing that 19% of trainers thought that their current FD had poor time management skills.[52]

Poor time management could be more than a case of simply running late and could include undue pressure from your ES or the practice receptionist. Table 2.5 lists some common causes of poor time management and their possible remedies.

TABLE 2.5 Common causes of poor time management

Cause	Remedy
Limited work ethic of FD	Observe how other GDPs work (such as your ES) and consider replicating their work rate and professionalism
Overly ambitious treatment within appointment time	Keep appointments to performing pre-scheduled treatments only
Time pressures resulting from unrealistic appointment duration	Work with your ES to set an appointment duration for typical treatment and ensure that the receptionist is also aware
Unscheduled appointment demand	Sometimes there can be pressure from the receptionist to see patients for emergency care. Learn when to say no, as it is often safer not to see a patient than to rush his or her care

It is important for you to have an open dialogue with your ES regarding how long you need for each clinical procedure, and all members of the team should be aware of this, including the practice receptionist. There is also an element of professionalism required here, because it is tempting to overestimate how long you may need for an appointment so you can afford an unscheduled break, which would obviously not be fair to yourself or your training practice. There is a general expectation for you to need less scheduled time for

52 Gilmour A, Jones R, Bullock AD. *Dental Foundation Trainers' Expectations of a Dental Graduate.* Final Report. Cardiff: Wales Deanery/Cardiff University; 2012. p. 14.

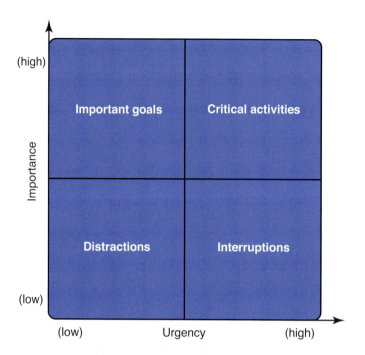

FIGURE 2.1 Graphical representation of the relationship between Urgent and Important activities

clinical procedures during the course of the year as your performance of skills becomes more intuitive.

The efficient management of time and resources on a daily basis is a COPDEND curriculum competency[53] that you are expected to demonstrate during FT. The Time-Management Matrix[54] (*see* Figure 2.1) is a powerful way of thinking about how you spend your time. Using it helps you overcome the natural tendency to focus on interesting activities, so that you can keep clear enough time to focus on what's really important.

'Not Urgent and Not Important' activities are considered to be distractions to be avoided if possible – for instance, surfing the internet in the workplace environment. 'Not Urgent but Important' activities are those that will help you achieve your professional goals, such as project work during the year. Make sure that you have plenty of time to do these things properly, so that they do

53 Committee of Postgraduate Dental Deans and Directors UK (COPDEND). *Interim Dental Foundation Training Curriculum & Assessment Framework Guidance 2013–2014*. Oxford: COPDEND; 2013. Management & leadership domain, ¶1 (1).

54 Covey SR. *The 7 Habits of Highly Effective People: powerful lessons in personal change*. New York: Simon & Schuster; 1989. p. 146.

not become urgent. 'Urgent and Not Important' activities are considered to be interruptions that stop you achieving your goals, and prevent you from completing your work. Finally, 'Urgent and Important' activities are those that are considered critical and to which you should devote your time. You can avoid last-minute activities by planning ahead and avoiding procrastination, although crises cannot always be foreseen.

INDUCTION

The purpose of an induction programme is to help you to acclimatise to, and become integrated within, the practice environment. Given the volume of information that you will be exposed to and expected to remember when starting out, it is not uncommon for your induction to take several days, if not weeks. In fact, an induction programme is best delivered in slices within the first month through a combination of practical tasks and patient contact.

The main components of induction are orientation with the facilities and processes, and socialisation within the team. For many FDs, FT will be their first job, and the prospect of working with strangers as part of a team can be nerve-wracking. Box 2.1 shows the different areas that your ES may specifi-cally cover.

Educational Supervisors have differing approaches to how soon you should have patient contact. Just be sure that you are well prepared to start seeing patients, particularly given the long break between dental school and the start of FT. This is because seeing patients when you are unfamiliar with your clinical environment could be damaging to your confidence from the outset. Do not be afraid to inform your ES that you would like more time to acclimatise to your clinical environment or to rationalise complex informa-tion such as the NHS regulations.

 ACTION POINT! Which induction topics would you like to have explained to you by your ES within the first few weeks? Here's some suggestions to start you off:
- Dental equipment: how to use it
- Clinical record entries: where to write them
- NHS rules and regulations: what can or can't you offer to patients
- Referrals: where and how you can refer
- ....
- ....

BOX 2.1 Areas potentially covered at induction

Team	Facilities
Introduction to your team members	Practice and clinic layout
Roles of team members	Location of services (water mains, electricity mains and gas supply)
Shadowing your team members	Practice security
Referral policies (for additional or advanced mandatory services and internally to dental care professionals)	Opening and closing practice (alarm, compressor, mains, answerphone)
Staff meetings	Routine surgery procedures at start and end of session
	Surgery equipment use
	Reporting breakdowns and faults
	Protocol for stock control and ordering
	Location of emergency drugs and equipment
	Radiation protection – local rules
	Emergency X-ray malfunction procedure
	Mains switch, compressor, aspirator maintenance procedures
Clinical	**Administration**
Patient management	Health and safety policy
Clinical guidelines (such as NICE wisdom tooth extraction*)	COSHH (control of substances hazardous to health) folder
Safety equipment: glasses, gloves, mask, apron	Practice risk assessments
Exposing, developing and storing radiographs	Accident and incident reporting
Waste disposal procedure and policy	Sickness reporting policy
Syringes – loading and unloading	Completing NHS forms
Disinfection and decontamination process	Medical history forms
Recall policy (NICE guidelines[†])	Record keeping (practice software)
Medical emergencies and basic life support (BLS) training	Appointment management
Practising procedures on extracted teeth	Practice information leaflet
Practice audits	Complaints procedure
	Holiday booking procedure
	Time and location of weekly tutorials
	Fire drill procedure
	Equal opportunities policy

* NICE Technology Appraisal Guidance – No.1. *Guidance on the Extraction of Wisdom Teeth*; March 2000.
[†] NICE Clinical Guideline 19. *Dental Recall: recall interval between routine dental examinations*; October 2004.

PRE-START CHECKLIST

Before your first day in practice you should:

Task	Completed?
Have your GDC registration number and indemnity cover in place	
Have already completed all forms for inclusion onto NHS England's national dental performers list and have either been included, or are close to being included	
Have already completed your Educational Agreement and the Foundation (employment) Contract with your ES	
Have already visited your ES at the practice to meet the team, understand your commute, and so forth	
Be in possession of several uniforms to wear after having discussing this with your ES	
Know your working hours, including what time you are expected to attend on Day 1	
Have your log-in details for e-PDP (if you have problems, contact Smile-On)	
Have your scheme study day programme	
Have your P45 ready to give to your ES or practice owner, or alternatively the information requested of you within a 'starter checklist'	

FIRST-WEEK CHECKLIST

Within your first week in practice you should:

Task	Completed?
Log in to e-PDP (if you have problems, contact Smile-On) to complete your personal details	
Jointly complete the Educational Agreement section of e-PDP with your ES	
Complete the 'Week 1: Clinical Experience Log' on e-PDP	
Understand the practice's system of record keeping, receiving some IT software training if computerised	
Become familiar with using the equipment and materials in the surgery you shall be working in	
Know the precise location and how to access medical emergency drugs and equipment	
Read and ask questions about the practice's policies and procedures	
Understand the various NHS administrative forms used in practice (FP17, FP17DC, FP17PR, FP17RN)	
Understand the role and responsibilities of each member of the team, possibly spending time with each member to shadow them	

Task	Completed?
Complete ESPR 1, with your ES recording this on e-PDP	
Complete D-CbD 1, with your ES recording this on e-PDP	
Complete 'Week 1: Reflection' on e-PDP	
Complete the 'Week 1: Weekly Log' on e-PDP	
Speak with your ES or practice owner about tax (Pay As You Earn, or PAYE) and National Insurance (NI) Also establish when and how you are likely to get paid	

GETTING IN THE 'FLOW'

During the first few months of FT, FDs are commonly anxious about perform-ing most clinical procedures, including for instance taking radiographs and impressions, which can be challenging as your skills are usually less advanced having been left dormant since after graduation. As you practise these clinical procedures more often your skills will improve and the procedures should prove less of a challenge to you. At this stage of FT, continually performing the same procedures can become boring as they would become less of a challenge for your higher skill-set. To avoid becoming bored during the year, you must encounter new procedures which pose a greater challenge in order to stretch your current skill-set, thereby enabling you to work in that optimal zone between anxiety and boredom (*see* Figure 2.2). You will then be, as Mihály Csíkszentmihályi asserts,[55] in the flow, whereby:

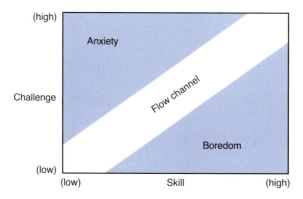

FIGURE 2.2 Graphical representation of the optimal operating zone between anxiety and boredom

55   Csíkszentmihályi M. *Beyond Boredom and Anxiety: experiencing flow in work and play*. 25th Anniversary Edition. San Francisco, CA: Jossey-Bass; 2000.

Every action, movement, and thought follows inevitably from the previous one …. Your whole being is involved, and you're using your skills to the utmost.

PREDICTING PERFORMANCE

It is difficult to predict your clinical performance during FT based on your academic track record or national recruitment ranking since they specifically exclude an assessment of your clinical skills. This is consistent with evidence that shows that the link between academic record and clinical performance is not clearly defined.[56] Therefore, unless you had performed a significantly greater range or amount of clinical procedures than other undergraduates, it is likely that you would have approximately the same baseline clinical competence as other FDs at the start of the year.

THE CONFIDENCE–COMPETENCE MATRIX

As an undergraduate you would have had to learn complex new skills, and therefore almost certainly would have experienced a fleeting dip in confidence when you realised that you needed more practice in order to move forward. It is probably during this time that you felt most discouraged that your motivation for learning new skills is tested. The best way of explaining this phenomenon during FT is by mapping out your levels of learning onto a graph that plots your competence in a particular skill against your confidence in delivering that skill (*see* Figure 2.3).

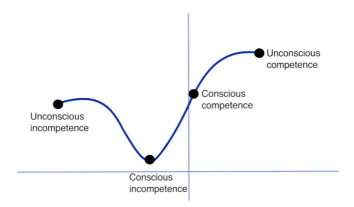

FIGURE 2.3 Levels of learning, plotting confidence against competence

---

56 Smithers S, Catano VM, Cunningham DP. What predicts performance in Canadian dental schools? *J Dent Educ.* 2004; **68**(6): 596–613.

FDs travel through various levels of learning[57] during the FT programme for each new skill they acquire.

- *Months 1–2.* You start off at a baseline confidence level represented by *unconscious incompetence* when you have no awareness of what you do not know. After being gently introduced to the clinical environment this is when you feel, with blissful ignorance, that you are surviving FT. Spending too long in the *unconscious incompetence* stage of the learning journey increases the risk of adverse incidents. The best tools you can use to leave this stage are self-reflection, to help identify precisely what you do not know so well, and self-directed learning.
- *Months 3–5.* Your confidence level then drops down to the *conscious incompetence* level when you start seeing more patients, and you suddenly become aware of the skills and knowledge that you still need to develop. This 'dip' is inevitable and must be passed through, but what you should not do at this stage is try to avoid procedures involving skills you have not yet developed.
- *Months 6–10.* The next step is when you can perform the various stages of a skill, reliably and at will. Your confidence at performing the skill will increase but you still need to actively think about whether you are performing the various stages of the skill correctly. As the gradient illustrates, the transition from *conscious incompetence* to *conscious competence* is generally considered the most difficult. The best way to move to the next level is to practise the skill.
- *Months 11–12.* You start to demonstrate flashes of *unconscious competence*, when the skill becomes so practised that it becomes second nature. As the matrix shows, this is where your confidence and competence are at their peak. Teaching and explaining to others how you perform the skill may, however, still prove difficult.
- *Post Month 12.* Not illustrated on the matrix is the final level of *reflective competence*, during which you develop the ability to instinctively reflect and adjust the skill to new contexts. This is when you are able to comfortably explain to others exactly how you perform the skill.

The *Dunning–Kruger effect*[58] is the finding that the poorest performers are the least aware of their own incompetence. Incompetent performers *overestimate*

---

57   Robinson WL. Conscious competency: the mark of a competent instructor. *Personnel Journal.* 1974; 53: 538–9.

58   Kruger J, Dunning D. Unskilled and unaware of it: how difficulties in recognizing one's own incompetence lead to inflated self-assessments. *J Pers Soc Psychol.* 1999 Dec; 77(6): 1121–34.

how good they are at carrying out a task, with their perceived performance outstripping their actual performance. This gap is reversed for competent performers, who commonly underestimate themselves, whereby their actual performance outstrips their perceived performance.

Research has identified overestimation as being distinct from other types of overconfidence,[59] which can be applied to dentistry as follows:

- *overprecision* – excessive certainty in the accuracy of our clinical knowledge base
- *overestimation* – the belief in our ability to carry out a clinical procedure or task
- *overplacement* – the belief that we are better than our peers at carrying out a clinical procedure or task.

> . . . all I know is that I know nothing.
>
> —Socrates (469–399 BC)

MINDING THE GAPS

As classified by Miller,[60] methods of assessment can be classified in a model depicted as a pyramid (*see* Figure 5.1). By climbing up the pyramid, the learner passes through successive stages, as outlined in Figure 2.4.

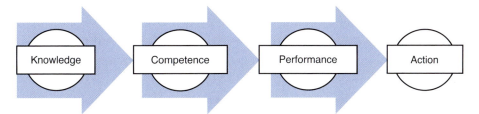

FIGURE 2.4 Progress through Miller's pyramid

As a *safe beginner*, chances are that you would have already demonstrated the required degree of knowledge and how to apply this knowledge under specific conditions. Therefore, you would have already made the leap over the gap between *knowledge* and *competence*. In the FT year the desired outcome of

59 Mannes AE, Moore DA. A behavioral demonstration of overconfidence in judgment. *Psychol Sci.* 2013; **24**(7): 1190–7.

60 Miller GE. The assessment of clinical skills/competence/performance. *Acad Med.* 1990; **65**(9 Suppl.): S63–7.

training is for you to demonstrate clinical competence and therefore for you to leap the gap between *competence* and *performance*. Once you do this you will have successfully applied your knowledge to treating patients in the clinical setting. Indeed, this is what the role of your ES and FTPD are, to help close the gap between your *competence* and your *performance*.

Making the final leap from *performance* to everyday *action* is more difficult because this is not achieved by showing others that you can apply your knowledge but actually doing what you know when nobody is assessing you. Transferring what you know to what you do when treating patients is not a simple process, as dentistry is not an exact science and no two patients are alike. Therefore, leaping the final gap will forever be under the dark cloud of the threat of consequences, such as patient complaints, if you do not achieve what you set out. Just try to remember that good patient communication skills and being able to learn from your errors will act as a parachute when making that final leap.

> *Integrity is doing the right thing, even when no one is watching.*
>
> —CS Lewis (1898–1963)

MANAGEMENT AND LEADERSHIP

One of the domains that you are expected to demonstrate within this year is management and leadership. Although 'management' and 'leadership' are terms that are used interchangeably, they are in fact discrete entities. Whereas management describes a collection of processes that help an entity, such as your practice, to perform in a predictable way, leadership involves taking that entity into the future, identifying opportunity as well as risk. It can be daunting for you, as an FD at practice level, to be expected to take the lead, but inside of the four walls of the surgery that you work within you are in fact the team leader. Just as with any team, there needs to be a leader who paints a vision, enabling team members to realise that vision.

Teaching and learning

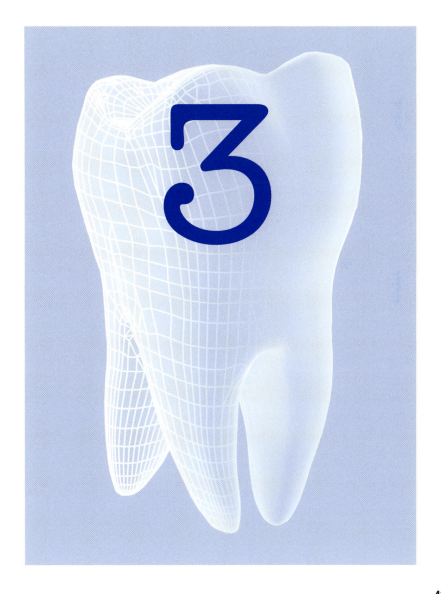

Teaching does not take place in isolation; it is linked both to developing a curriculum and to assessment. These three activities, along with a method of quality assurance, make up the educational paradigm (*see* Figure 3.1).

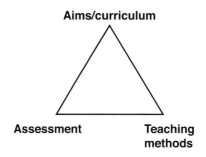

FIGURE 3.1 Educational paradigm

Assessment drives learning, providing an indication of your performance against the expected ability of an FD at the equivalent stage. It also helps the teacher to evaluate his or her teaching, identifying where this can be improved and helping to develop the curriculum defined for you.

Curriculum, derived from the Latin for track, has been defined[61] as '*an educational plan that spells out which goals and objectives should be achieved, which topics should be covered and which methods are to be used for learning, teaching and evaluation.*' Your curriculum therefore refers not only to the COPDEND Dental Foundation Training Curriculum but also to your bespoke learning needs identified from a learning needs assessment conducted by your ES at the beginning of FT.

Your ES and FTPD will most likely teach you using a combination the following methods:
- *Didactic* – telling you information
- *Socratic* – asking you questions to engage you in a dialogue to explore your understanding in more depth
- *Heuristic* – encouraging you to discover and therefore learn something yourself, such as problem-based learning
- *Counselling* – exploring your feelings and insights in order to help unblock emotions blocking your learning.

Linking learning into practice is desirable in FT, and as skills and knowledge are acquired, it is paramount that you return the demonstration of a learned

61 Wojtczak A. Institute for International Medical Education. *Glossary of Medical Education Terms.* Available at: www.iime.org/glossary.htm (accessed November 2013).

skill. The primary purpose of 'return demonstration' is to verify your ability to perform the skill, and to experience progress in your understanding and application of the education.

ONE-TO-ONE TEACHING

The training practice environment gives rise to experiencing one-to-one teaching between you and your ES. This method of teaching differs considerably from lecture and other group-based teaching methods that you may have experienced at undergraduate level. One-to-one teaching is underpinned by the trust that you build with your ES. As a result of you being more closely observed, you cannot easily hide your weaknesses from the teacher, since your skills, knowledge, reactions and opinions are all magnified. Rather than thinking of this as intrusive, it is actually a very helpful tool to identify what you need to learn, thereby helping your teacher to customise his or her teaching in order to accurately address your learning needs. In fact, Ausubel *et al.*[62] have suggested that the secret of education is to find out what the learner already knows and to teach accordingly.

Learning in the clinical environment provides a focus on real problems in the context of dental practice, although time pressures and competing patient demands can often prove challenging. This is why at least an hour a week is dedicated to one-to-one teaching with your ES. Tutorials are the backbone of in-practice teaching and they usually take place during the working day, in protected time (not within your lunch hour). There are different approaches to delivering tutorials and these may involve:

- reviewing e-PDP outstanding tasks
- discussing how learning outcomes from the previous study day have been applied to practice
- discussing any complex cases
- discussing operational or administrative issues (equipment, materials, payment, etc.)
- obtaining assistance with project work such as the FT portfolio of evidence and audit
- reviewing case presentation cases
- teaching of a tutorial topic
- conducting a workplace-based assessment (WPBA)

---

62   Ausubel D, Novak J, Hanesian H. *Educational Psychology: a cognitive view*. 2nd ed. New York, NY: Holt, Rinehart, & Winston; 1978.

- agreeing next week's tutorial subject and any preparatory work
- completing the tutorial reflection section on e-PDP.

Tutorial topics ought to be agreed between you and your ES in advance, to be the most relevant. For instance, if you are struggling with extractions it would be prudent to cover oral surgery in the proceeding tutorial. Once agreed, the method of learning within the tutorial could be:
- carrying out a clinical procedure on a patient together
- asking you to present a topic to the ES, after having researched it, or
- speaking about and reflecting upon particular cases of difficulty.

> **ACTION POINT!** To get the most benefit out of your weekly tutorials get into the habit of keeping a notepad to jot down any questions you have during the course of the week. You can then bring up these questions with your ES during your next tutorial.

ONE-TO-ONE FEEDBACK

One-to-one supervision and assessment in practice ultimately leads to receiving feedback based on the observation of your performance by your ES. Accepting and providing effective feedback in a manner that motivates and encourages learning is a COPDEND curriculum competency[63] that you are expected to demonstrate during FT. Feedback will generally be given to you immediately after your performance, such as in an A'DEP'T, in a factual and targeted way. As evidenced by Smoll[64] 'knowledge of results' feedback is most beneficial when there is some quantitative nature attached to it – for instance, the clearance height required in a crown preparation.

In a randomised controlled trial conducted by Boehler *et al.*,[65] it was found that clinical students showed greater improvement in the performance of a task when given constructive feedback than when given praise alone. This implies that what we like to hear and what we need to hear in order to advance our clinical skills may be very different. It is important that you react positively to all feedback received, otherwise critical feedback may act to damage

---

63 Committee of Postgraduate Dental Deans and Directors UK (COPDEND). *Interim Dental Foundation Training Curriculum & Assessment Framework Guidance 2013–2014.* Oxford: COPDEND; 2013. Management & leadership domain, ¶4 (7).

64 Smoll FL. Effects of precision of information feedback upon acquisition of a motor skill. *Research Quarterly.* 1972; **43**: 489–93.

65 Boehler ML, Rogers DA, Schwind CJ, *et al.* An investigation of medical student reactions to feedback: a randomised controlled trial. *Med Educ.* 2006; **40**(8): 746–9.

your self-esteem, while compliments may risk making you complacent. It is important to incorporate feedback into actions entered into the Personal Development Plan section of e-PDP – to add an item, click 'Add PDP item'.

Feedback is not merely praise or approval but, rather, a realistic appraisal of your performance that can help to identify your strengths and weaknesses. Try to respond to feedback by reflecting rather than being tempted to offer counterarguments to defend your thoughts and actions. Feedback allows you to validate your own assessment of performance to ensure that you are being realistic with your own self-reflection.

 TIP! By definition, 'feedback' places the emphasis on past performance, whereas 'feedforward' is about being aware of your performance in the present and is based upon an anticipated result, acting to remedy the cause of poor technique as opposed to its symptoms.

STUDY DAY PROGRAMME

Clause 17.8 of the Foundation Contract outlines a requirement for you to attend all study day (otherwise known as day release) courses, with clause 16.2 identifying that there are approximately 30 study days within the programme for the year. The study day programme is arranged by the FTPD, with the assistance of an administrator and along with in-practice tutorials, aims to cover the nationally agreed competencies outlined within the COPDEND Dental Foundation Training Curriculum (*see* Chapter 4).

Study day teaching is considered as 'small group teaching', as it involves the teaching of a group of FDs within a scheme or patch. Traditionally the size of a scheme has been 12–14 FDs, but there is currently a growing approach to varying this group size. A balance must be struck between a larger group, where there is a greater pool of talent and experience available for solving problems, and a smaller group, enabling greater participation from each learner.

At study days there is generally less emphasis on FDs 'soaking up' the learning through lectures and more emphasis on learning activities. This is because studies have shown that student recall of facts can be improved with interaction and activity.[66] The content of the study day programme for each scheme tends to vary according to the learning needs of the FDs within that scheme. Study days are usually based at a specified postgraduate dental education cen-

---

66 Bligh DA. *What's the Use of Lectures?* San Francisco, CA: Jossey-Bass; 2000.

tre, but there may be opportunities where study days are held off-site, such as when attending lectures at local or national dental conferences, where you can network with FDs from other schemes. Although there are a number of interesting dental activities and conferences available to attend, these can only form part of your study day programme if your FTPD deems the teaching to be aligned to the COPDEND curriculum competencies.

As the syllabi for the Membership of the Faculty of Dental Surgery (MFDS) and Membership of the Joint Dental Faculties (MJDF) examinations are aligned to the COPDEND Dental Foundation Training Curriculum, it is unlikely that you would have a study day dedicated towards preparing you for the examination, as theoretically all study days held will cover the syllabi. You generally need to fund your own travel to and from study days, but there is scope to claim for some travel and subsistence by completing and submitting an FP84 claim form.

NON-STUDY DAY COURSES

Outside of your study day programme there is nothing preventing you from attending other postgraduate dental education courses, so long as they do not impinge on your FT commitments. There are many sources of postgraduate dental courses that are CPD verifiable, including your LETB, British Dental Association (BDA) branch section and local dental committee (LDC). It is generally advisable not to enrol onto a course requiring a specific level of time commitment, as this may limit the time you can dedicate towards completing FT requirements and preparing for interviews.

An understanding of the importance of the team management of medical emergencies, and being able to facilitate such an approach, is a COPDEND curriculum competency[67] that you are expected to demonstrate during FT. Also, in your e-PDP Clinical Experience Log there is an expectation that you would have had BLS and medical emergencies training during your FT year. This is often arranged by your training practice and involves the entire dental team, but if not you can still access BLS and medical emergencies training through your LETB.

---

67   Committee of Postgraduate Dental Deans and Directors UK (COPDEND). *Interim Dental Foundation Training Curriculum & Assessment Framework Guidance 2013–2014*. Oxford: COPDEND; 2013. Clinical domain, ¶4 (8).

ACTION POINT! Familiarise yourself with the medical emergency drugs and equipment in your practice. Also read the Resuscitation Council UK's *Medical Emergencies and Resuscitation: standards for clinical practice and training for dental practitioners and dental care professionals in general dental practice.** Available at: www.resus.org.uk/pages/MEdental.pdf

* Resuscitation Council (UK). *Medical Emergencies and Resuscitation: standards for clinical practice and training for dental practitioners and dental care professionals in general dental practice, Revised 2012.* London: Resuscitation Council (UK); 2012.

EXPERIENTIAL LEARNING

As the name suggests, the experiential learning theory, proposed by David Kolb,[68] involves learning from experience. 'Concrete experience' provides the information that serves as a basis for reflection, from which we can form 'abstract generalisations'. Reflection is to stand back from the concrete experience and consider what it meant, how it relates to other past experiences and how you felt (*see* Chapter 5). We can then use our generalisations, obtained through reflection, to develop new theories, which we can then actively test. Through the 'active experimentation' of our ideas, we can consider what we will do differently the next time we encounter a similar experience, therefore cycling back to the beginning of the process.

Every learning process, however, does not necessarily begin with encountering a concrete experience. Instead, each person must choose which learning mode will work best, based upon the given situation. For instance, some of us learn a new clinical skill best by reflecting upon observing somebody else perform that skill, others learn more abstractly through textbooks, while yet others learn best through performing the skill themselves.

HONEY AND MUMFORD'S LEARNING STYLES QUESTIONNAIRE

People do not learn in the same way. Developed by Peter Honey and Alan Mumford[69] and based upon the work of Kolb, learning styles group common ways that people learn. The four distinct learning styles are as follows.
1. *Activists*: learn best by being thrown in the deep end with a difficult task, and they like to lead discussions.

---

68 Kolb DA. *Experiential Learning.* Englewood Cliffs, NJ: Prentice Hall; 1984.
69 Honey P, Mumford A. *Manual of Learning Styles.* London: P Honey; 1982.

2. *Theorists*: learn best when they can question reasoning and when they are in structured situations with a clear purpose.
3. *Pragmatists*: learn best when the net benefit of learning a task is explained, and when they have the chance to try out techniques with feedback (e.g. role-playing).
4. *Reflectors*: learn best by observing others at work, and when they are given an opportunity to think about what has happened and what they have learned.

To understand your particular learning style, Honey and Mumford have developed a Learning Styles Questionnaire that, following completion, allows you to identify your preferred learning style. Some people may find that they have a dominant style of learning with far less use of the other styles. Others may find that they use different styles in different circumstances. There is no right or wrong mix. Your preferred learning style guides the way you learn and changes the way in which you internally represent experiences and recall information. By identifying and understanding your preferred learning style, your FT experience can be tailored to use learning techniques better suited to you, which will improve the speed and quality of your learning.

Honey and Mumford have built a typology of learning styles around the experiential learning cycle, which identifies individual preferences for each stage (*see* Figure 3.2), but to effectively learn you must complete all stages of the cycle.

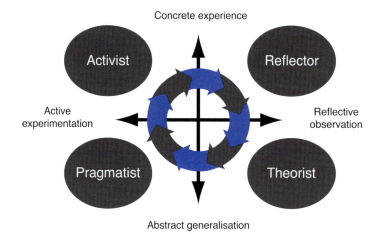

FIGURE 3.2 Typology of learning styles around the experiential learning cycle

ACTION POINT! Why not explore how you learn best by attempting Honey and Mumford's Learning Styles Questionnaire? You or your ES can access this at: www.peterhoney.com

MEMORY

Learning any new skill can be difficult, and it starts with the use of our working memory to temporarily store new information. For learning a clinical skill, this will involve breaking down and remembering each action of the procedure into bite-sized chunks. However, the working memory store has limited space and the information can be unstable – for instance, a sudden distraction may lose the information and you have to start again from scratch. Once practised enough, the skill will become so ingrained that it is almost automatically performed, which is when we use our procedural memory to store this information on a long-term basis. Procedural memory is a memory of motor, perceptual or cognitive skills and is therefore responsible for you knowing how to 'do' things. Let's take the example of tying a simple interrupted suture. Following adequate practice, although it may become easy enough to demonstrate the skill to others, explaining each action can prove more difficult. Therefore, we often need to deconstruct (or de-learn) a skill in order to correct fundamental errors of understanding, before we reconstruct (or relearn) the same skill.

As contended by Malcolm Gladwell,[70] the key to success in any field is, to a large extent, a matter of deliberately practising a specific task for a total of around 10 000 hours. It is important that deliberate practice takes place in different contexts, because even with 10 000 hours' practice on cutting crowns in phantom heads, you will not be guaranteed a predictable outcome working within the changeable conditions of the oral cavity.

To commit learning to memory, Piotr Wozniak has theorised,[71] there is an ideal moment to practise what you have learned. Practise too soon and you waste your time; practise too late and you will most likely forget the material and will need to relearn it. The right time to practise is just at the moment that you are about to forget it. The SuperMemo learning programme advocates that we forget exponentially, with your chance of recalling a given skill declining over time according to a predictable pattern (*see* Figure 3.3). When

70 Gladwell M. *Outliers: the story of success*. 1st ed. New York, NY: Little, Brown and Company; 2008.
71 Wozniak PA, Biedalak K. The SuperMemo method: optimization of learning. *Informatyka*. 1992; **10**: 1–9.

your chance of recalling a new skill drops to 90%, you should refresh your memory of it at the following intervals: 1, 10, 30 and 60 days afterwards.

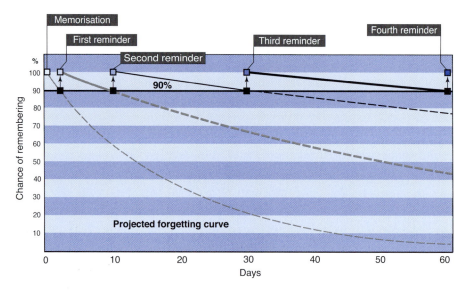

FIGURE 3.3 The SuperMemo learning program

LIGHT BULBS

In a study conducted by the Stanford University School of Medicine,[72] researchers used images of the brain of those listening to short symphonies by the composer William Boyce to look at how the brain makes sense of events. Having a mismatch between what listeners *anticipate* hearing from memory versus what they *actually* hear – such as an unrelated chord following an ongoing harmony pattern – triggers ventral regions of the brain akin to a light bulb being switched on. Once activated, those regions of the brain identify the unrelated chord as *different* with distinct boundaries. If our brains arrange learnt practical skills in the same way as music, then for those *compe-tent* in performing a clinical procedure, a light bulb should automatically be switched on each time the clinical procedure is performed incorrectly; thereby identifying precisely what needs to be corrected.

---

72 Sridharansend D, Levitin DJ, Chafe CH, *et al.* Neural dynamics of event segmentation in music: converging evidence for dissociable ventral and dorsal networks. *Neuron.* 2007; **55**(3): 521–32.

Curriculum

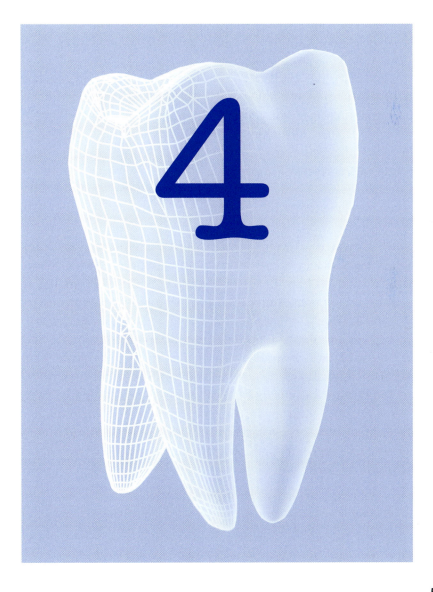

At undergraduate level you would have needed to satisfy a curriculum published by the GDC: *The First Five Years.*[73] In 2012 this was succeeded by *Preparing for Practice,*[74] which describes the outcomes that individuals must demonstrate by the end of their training, in order to register with the GDC. More specifically, *Preparing for Practice* divides the skills required of new registrants into four discrete domains.

1. *Clinical*: the range of skills required to deliver direct care, where registrants interact with patients, and also the essential technical skills, carried out in the absence of patients which support their care, for example, by dental technicians
2. *Communication*: the skills involved in effectively interacting with patients, their representatives, the public and colleagues and recording appropriate information to inform patient care
3. *Professionalism*: the knowledge, skills and attitudes/behaviours required to practise in an ethical and appropriate way, putting patients' needs first and promoting confidence in the dental team
4. *Management and Leadership*: the skills and knowledge required to work effectively as a dental team, manage their own time and resources and contribute to professional practices.

These have been aligned to the four domains contained within the COPDEND UK Dental Foundation Training Curriculum.[75] The four domains are interlinked, as shown in Figure 4.1 with the clinical, communication and management and leadership domains 'running through' the professionalism domain.

Within each domain, individual competency statements are grouped within themes known as 'major competencies'. Each of the major competencies also contain further specific, supporting 'minor competencies' that describe the skills and attributes expected of the FD. Therefore, to successfully complete FT you are expected to successfully demonstrate each of the documented competencies. To ensure that this is achieved, all teaching and assessment tools are mapped to the competencies. The Interim Curriculum and Assessment Framework Guidance for Dental Foundation Training has been developed to allow you to identify what outcomes are expected to have been achieved by the end of FT.

73   GDC. *The First Five Years: the undergraduate dental curriculum.* 3rd ed. (interim). London: GDC; 2008.
74   GDC. *Preparing for Practice: dental team learning outcomes for registration.* London: GDC; 2012.
75   COPDEND. *A Curriculum for UK Dental Foundation Programme Training.* 2007. Available at: www.copdend.org/data/files/Foundation/Dental%20Foundation%20Programme%20Curriculum.pdf (accessed November 2013).

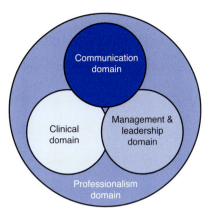

FIGURE 4.1 Interrelation between the four domains

The COPDEND UK Dental Foundation Training Curriculum[76] was originally designed to encompass 2 years of Dental Foundation Training. As this is no longer the case, COPDEND has outlined their intention to formally revise the curriculum to best meet 'the contemporary needs of new dental graduates in the critical period of transition to assured and proficient independent NHS practice'.[77]

Although outlining each minor competency is outwith the scope of this book, reference has been made to minor competencies throughout the content of this book where relevant. Table 4.1 lists an example of a minor competency belonging to each major competency and domain along with a summary of how it can be evidenced together with the tools used to assess it.[78]

76   COPDEND. *A Curriculum for UK Dental Foundation Programme Training.* Available at: www.copdend. org/data/files/Foundation/Dental%20Foundation%20Programme%20Curriculum.pdf (accessed November 2013).

77   Committee of Postgraduate Dental Deans and Directors UK (COPDEND). *Interim Dental Foundation Training Curriculum & Assessment Framework Guidance 2013–2014.* Oxford: COPDEND; 2013. p. 2.

78   Ibid.

TABLE 4.1 Methods used to assess various competencies

Domain	Major competency	Minor competency	Examples of evidence considered	Tools used to assess
Clinical	Patient Examination and Diagnosis	Can describe the investigations and assessment processes required prior to general anaesthesia	Observation in practice Tutorial or discussion e-Learning or lecture attendance	D-CbD
Clinical	Treatment Planning & Patient Management	Understands which items of treatment fall within NHS regulations and those which do not, and can discuss the consequences of this with the patient in a manner he or she can understand	Observation in practice Tutorial or discussion e-Learning or study day attendance Feedback from clinical team Patient feedback	A'DEP'T, PAQ and Multi-Source Feedback
Clinical	Health Promotion & Disease Prevention	Can describe in appropriate detail the health risks of substances such as tobacco and alcohol on oral health, and provide the patient with appropriate advice	Tutorial or discussion Simulation (study days) Observation in practice	A'DEP'T and trainer record in e-PDP following review of evidence
Clinical	Medical & Dental Emergencies	Can demonstrate a thorough understanding of potential drug interactions and side effects, and manage situations appropriately when they occur	Observation in practice Tutorial or discussion Feedback from clinical team and other health professionals	A'DEP'T, D-CbD and Multi-Source Feedback and trainer record in e-PDP following review of evidence

Domain	Major competency	Minor competency	Examples of evidence considered	Tools used to assess
Clinical	Anaesthesia Sedation, Pain & Anxiety Control	Can demonstrate, to an appropriate standard, the ability to use suitable behavioural, psychological and interpersonal techniques for the relief of fear and anxiety	Observation in practice e-Learning or lecture attendance Feedback from dental team Patient feedback Tutorial or discussion	A'DEP'T, D-CbD and PAQ
Clinical	Periodontal Therapy & Management of Soft Tissues	The conservative management of gingival recession	Observation in practice	A'DEP'T and D-CbD
Clinical	Hard & Soft Tissue Surgery	Can describe in appropriate detail the principles and techniques involved in the surgical placement of dental implants	Tutorial or discussion e-Learning or study day attendance	D-CbD
Clinical	Non-surgical Management of the Hard & Soft Tissues of the Head & Neck	Can demonstrate to an appropriate standard the ability to recognise and anticipate the potential drug interactions that may occur between medications prescribed by the patient's doctor and those used in dental practice	Tutorial or discussion Review of clinical records e-Learning or lecture attendance Observation in practice	A'DEP'T and D-CbD
Clinical	Management of the Developing Dentition	Can demonstrate appropriate knowledge and understanding of how to formulate and implement a plan to provide space maintenance when required	Tutorial or discussion Document review (treatment plans)	D-CbD and trainer record in e-PDP following review of evidence

Domain	Major competency	Minor competency	Examples of evidence considered	Tools used to assess
Clinical	Restoration of Teeth	Can demonstrate modern restorative concepts around Minimally Invasive Techniques	Observation in practice Tutorial or discussion e-Learning or study day attendance	A'DEP'T and D-CbD
Clinical	Replacement of Teeth	Can demonstrate to an appropriate standard the ability to prescribe to, and communicate with, the dental laboratory accurately, and assess the quality of the work completed by laboratory technicians	Review of clinical records or documents Feedback from professionals Tutorial or discussion	Trainer record in e-PDP following review of evidence
Communication	Patient & Family	Listens effectively and is responsive to non-verbal cues	Observation in practice Feedback from patients Feedback from dental team Simulation	A'DEP'T, PAQ and Multi-Source Feedback
Communication	Clinical Team & Peers	Understands the need for and can organise and facilitate team training events	Observation or review event	Trainer record in e-PDP following review of evidence
Communication	Other Professionals	Is able to explain the advantages of association with professional bodies and peer groups	Tutorial or discussion Study day attendance	Trainer report in e-PDP following review of evidence
Professionalism	Ethics	Respects and values diversity and interacts with patients, staff, peers and the general public without discrimination	Feedback from patients and team Tutorial or discussion e-Learning or study day attendance	PAQ, Multi-Source Feedback

Domain	Major competency	Minor competency	Examples of evidence considered	Tools used to assess
Professionalism	Patients	Provides relevant and appropriate preventive education for each patient in a manner that he/she can understand	Observation in practice Feedback from patients and team	A'DEP'T and PAQ
Professionalism	Self	Understands the significance of practising while impaired by alcohol, other drugs, illness or injury and can describe the dangers associated with these situations	Tutorial or discussion	Trainer record in e-PDP following review of evidence
Professionalism	Clinical Team & Peers	Understands the dynamics of multi-professional working and how these can contribute to the delivery of quality patient care	Feedback from dental team and other health professionals	D-CbD and Multi-Source Feedback
Management & Leadership	Personal & Practice Organisation	Can demonstrate an understanding of the considerations to be made during the selection, care and maintenance of equipment for dental practice	Tutorial or discussion e-Learning or study day attendance	Trainer record in e-PDP following review of evidence
Management & Leadership	Legislative	Has up-to-date knowledge and understanding of discrimination legislation	Tutorial or discussion	In-practice written or online assessment
Management & Leadership	Financial	Can demonstrate, to an appropriate standard, an understanding of business management and development, including the ability to develop a business plan, the production of a cash flow analysis and a written proposal to a bank	Tutorial or discussion	Trainer record in e-PDP following review of evidence
Management & Leadership	Leadership and Training	Can demonstrate to an appropriate standard the ability to select, implement and evaluate the effectiveness of teaching strategies to facilitate others' learning	Tutorial or discussion e-Learning or study day attendance	Trainer report in e-PDP following review of evidence

READING POINT! You can access the COPDEND *Interim Dental Foundation Training Curriculum & Assessment Framework Guidance* at: www.copdend.org//data/files/Foundation/Interim%20DFT%20curriculum%202013-14.pdf

e-Portfolio

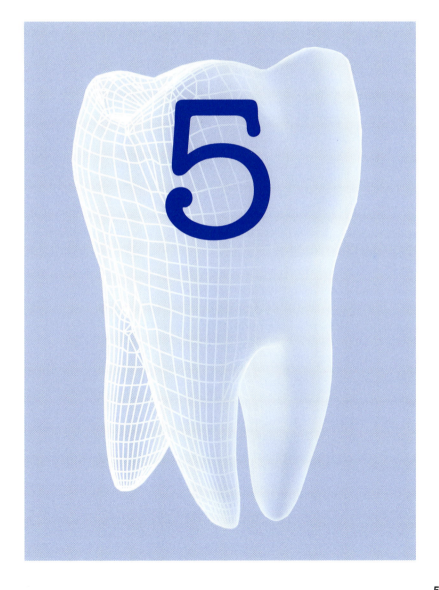

e-Portfolio (or e-PDP) is an online platform providing you with feedback on your performance and progress from your ES and FTPD, enabling you to triangulate this information with your own reflections on your practice. Clause 17.10 of the Foundation Contract requires you to maintain and complete e-PDP. You should be able to access e-PDP online, in surgery and during working hours within your training practice as stipulated in clause 16.1 of the Foundation Contract.

e-PDP is mapped to the COPDEND Dental Foundation Training Curriculum at the major competency level, and it enables three broad functions: (1) to monitor your progress, (2) to assess your performance and (3) to encourage you to reflect.

The 'Full learning plan' section on e-PDP lists all the activities that you are expected to complete throughout the year, specifically highlighting when they are due to be completed. The 'Current learning plan', however, lists activities still outstanding, as well as the current week's activities.

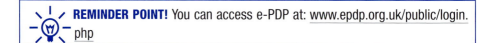

REMINDER POINT! You can access e-PDP at: www.epdp.org.uk/public/login.php

EDUCATIONAL AGREEMENT

The Educational Agreement section of e-PDP aims to personalise the obligations of both FD and ES. It is conducted through a joint exercise between you and your ES whereby you are required to discuss your ES's expectations of you, as well as your expectations of the ES, enabling you to highlight and document your obligations and responsibilities throughout the year. Suggestions for what you could write here include that you shall:
- respect patient confidentiality at all times
- attend the practice for the agreed hours
- determine personal learning needs with your ES
- complete reflections in a timely manner
- take an active part in weekly tutorials with your ES.

MONITORING

This is the gathering and recording of data to track your clinical and educational progress throughout FT and includes the following.

Clinical Experience Log

Although there is an expectation for you to have reached 'basic clinical skills' on graduation prior to commencing FT, there is no definitive consensus on what is defined as basic clinical skills, with the concept itself varying among dental schools. Therefore there is a need to ascertain your level of clinical experience, and confidence, prior to starting FT when you are required to complete the 'Week 1: Clinical Experience Log' before seeing any patients. The Clinical Experience Log must then be completed on a weekly basis throughout your training to identify the range and amount of clinical procedures you have performed. As this tool is used to monitor your experience it is essential that you accurately update the Clinical Experience Log contemporaneously.

Assessment Log

The Assessment Log is a record of the clinical focus of the different assessments carried out on your performance throughout training.

CPD and Education Log

The CPD and Education Log is a record of the verifiable and non-verifiable CPD, and other educational activities, undertaken during the programme. This may include study days, tutorials, seminars, conferences, and so forth.

Personal Development Plan

The Personal Development Plan (PDP) is used to monitor and record your learning needs as identified through assessments, reflections or other educational activities. To add an item to the Plan, click 'Add PDP item'.

ASSESSMENT

This refers to the quality measures used to determine your individual performance and mainly include WPBAs. As asserted by the Postgraduate Medical Education and Training Board, WPBAs are an assessment of your working practices based on what you actually do in the workplace and so are considered a more authentic assessment of your clinical performance than, say, Objective Structured Clinical Examinations.

A limitation of WPBAs, however, is that, on account of your performance being observed, it is arguably not a true indication what you actually 'do' in the workplace, but, rather, an indication of you 'showing how' something is done. This is because, as the *Hawthorne effect*[79] demonstrates, people alter their behaviour when being observed. What you 'do' when unobserved would be a truer indication of your actual performance, but the paradox is that this would be unable to be assessed, as it is not observed.

In Miller's 'pyramid of competence' model[80] (*see* Figure 5.1) a learner's *knowledge* is measured at the base of a pyramid followed by *competence* at the 'knows how' level; both are assessed under examination conditions with no reference to context. Meanwhile *performance* is measured at the 'shows how' level while *action* exists at the 'does' summit of the pyramid, assessed in more authentic real-time conditions. WPBAs exist near the top of the pyramid, as they assess *performance* within the context of different competencies of the clinical environment.

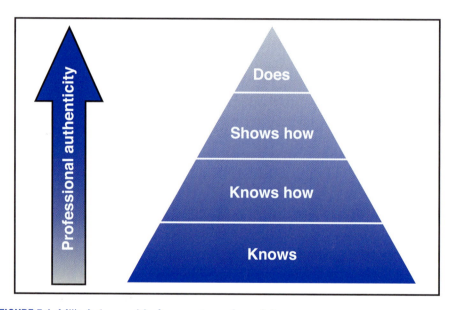

FIGURE 5.1 Miller's 'pyramid of competence' model

WPBAs are a formative assessment (i.e. not pass/fail) and are important, as they evidence your satisfactory progress throughout the FT programme, which may even be considered after you have completed the programme.

---

79   Roethlisberger FJ, Dickson WJ. *Management and the Worker: an account of a research program conducted by the Western Electric Company. Hawthorne Works, Chicago.* Harvard University Press; 1939.

80   Miller GE. The assessment of clinical skills/competence/performance. *Acad Med.* 1990; **65**(9 Suppl.): S63–7.

ESPR

ESPR assessments provide a structured way of assessing your ability within the first 4 weeks to confirm your *safe beginner* status (*see* Chapter 1). ESPRs involve your ES presenting procedures to you, and vice versa, enabling you to receive feedback. ESPRs also provide your ES with the opportunity to identify where your strengths and weaknesses lie, which may result in targeted remedial training if necessary.

TABLE 5.1 Details of the ESPR

Assessment type	WPBA
Number to be completed	Four within the first month
Assessor	ES
Standard compared against	That of a competent FD at this same early stage
How assessed	The assessor records his or her comments on your performance after discussion with you, and indicates whether the outcome of your performance is satisfactory for this stage in training or whether targeted training is required
Suitable activities to be assessed	Simple, clinical procedures such as the administration of effective local anaesthetic, the identification of caries, placement of rubber dam, taking an impression and the taking and interpreting of radiographs
Unsuitable activities to be assessed	Complex clinical procedures such as extractions
Satisfactory performance	If there are no major concerns about your ability to perform the procedures observed or if you would not directly benefit from some initial targeted training before continuing

A'DEP'T

A'DEP'Ts have been designed specifically for FT to record judgements on your performance following observation of a specific patient encounter or case. Ordinarily, the assessor gives you feedback promptly following your performance, at which point your insight into your performance will also be assessed.

TABLE 5.2 Details of the A'DEP'T

Assessment type	WPBA
Number to be completed	12 within the year
Assessor	11 assessed by the ES and 1 assessed by the FTPD
Standard compared against	That of a competent FD at the completion stage of FT
How assessed	The assessor judges performance and clinical decision-making across several broad areas on the basis of case presentation and any additional case notes available, using a 6-point scale ranging from 'needs improvement' to 'borderline' to 'acceptable' to 'above expectations'
Suitable activities to be assessed	Wide range of cases focusing on the competencies within all 11 clinical major competencies from the COPDEND Dental Foundation Training Curriculum
Satisfactory performance	Receiving no 'Needs Improvement' ratings, although such areas of performance can still be addressed and reassessed before the end of the post to provide evidence that progress has been made to a satisfactory level

D-CbD

D-CbD assessments involve you presenting a case to the assessor who then judges your performance and clinical decision-making on the basis of that presentation and any additional case notes and so forth available. Following your presentation the assessor will proceed to provide you with feedback on your performance, which ordinarily commences with the assessor asking you to reflect on your strengths and weaknesses regarding this case so that a judgement can be made on your insight. Once the D-CbD assessment form has been completed, with all ratings and feedback documented, the assessor will be able to discuss the case with you.

TABLE 5.3 Details of the D-CbD

Assessment type	WPBA
Number to be completed	12 within the year
Assessor	11 assessed by the ES and 1 assessed by the FTPD
Standard compared against	That of a competent FD at the completion stage of FT
How assessed	The assessor judges performance following a patient encounter, rating performance across several broad criteria against a 6-point scale ranging from 'needs improvement' to 'borderline' to 'acceptable' and to 'above expectations'

Suitable activities to be assessed	Wide range of cases focusing on the competencies within all 11 clinical major competencies from the COPDEND Dental Foundation Training Curriculum
Satisfactory performance	Receiving no 'Needs Improvement' ratings, although such areas of performance can still be addressed and reassessed before the end of the post to provide evidence that progress has been made to a satisfactory level

PAQ

The PAQ assessment involves you distributing at least 50 questionnaires to consecutive adult patients whom you have cared for over a 4-week period. Completed forms must remain anonymous and a minimum of 20 are required for reliable analysis.

TABLE 5.4 Details of the PAQ

Assessment type	Questionnaires
Number to be completed	50 responses by Week 23
Assessor	ES
Standard compared against	That of a competent FD at the completion stage of FT
How assessed	The assessor judges performance in various areas through the responses provided by patients across several areas including communication and professionalism
	Patients rate you against a 5-point scale ranging from 'strongly agree' to 'agree' to 'neither agree nor disagree' to 'disagree' and to 'strongly disagree', as well as entering any written comments
Suitable patients to complete questionnaires	All adult patients consecutively chosen within a 4-week period leading up to Week 23
Satisfactory performance	The absence of any 'strongly disagree' ratings or adverse comments from patients, although such areas of performance can still be addressed and reassessed before the end of the post to provide evidence that progress has been made to a satisfactory level

REFLECTION

This refers to the process of better understanding an experience to inform future action. Reflecting encourages you to think back over an incident using different perspectives (such as the perspective of your patient or dental nurse) to enhance deeper learning by identifying learning needs. Documenting all of this cements the process.

Schön[81] asserts that while the 'effective' reflective clinician recognises and explores confusing or unique events that occur during practice, the 'ineffective' clinician is confined to repetitive practice, neglecting opportunities to think about what he or she is doing. Providing an insight into your feelings is also a key part of the Gibbs[82] reflective cycle (*see* Figure 5.2).

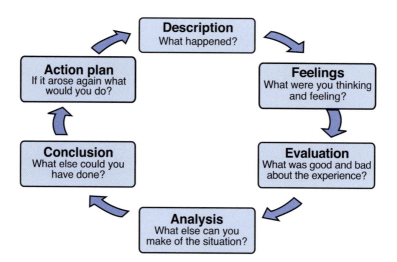

FIGURE 5.2 Gibbs reflective cycle

81   Schön D. *The Reflective Practitioner: how professionals think in action.* New York, NY: Basic Books; 1983.
82   Gibbs G. *Learning by Doing: a guide to teaching and learning methods.* Oxford: Further Education Unit, Oxford Polytechnic; 1988.

Reflection (in-practice)

TABLE 5.5 Details of the in-practice reflections

Number to be completed	19 within the year (weekly for the first 2 months, then on a monthly basis thereafter)
Assessor	ES and FTPD
How assessed	Each of the seven sections within the e-PDP reflection response is reviewed and comments provided
Suitable activities to be assessed	• Your progress towards achieving specific competencies within the COPDEND Dental Foundation Training Curriculum • A significant clinical case • A significant patient-related incident (i.e. difficulty placing rubber dam) • A significant team-related incident (i.e. disagreement with your dental nurse) • A significant professionalism-related incident (i.e. poor punctuality) • Progress towards a previously identified learning need • Study day course • Non-study day course • First 8 weeks
Satisfactory performance	All seven sections of the reflection response must be adequately completed, demonstrating active reflection

Table 5.6 outlines the seven items that need to be completed for each reflection as prompted by e-PDP.

TABLE 5.6 Areas to be completed for the in-practice reflection

1. Subject	Confirming the subject of the reflection
2. Date	Date relating to when you reflected upon the incident rather than of the incident
3. Details	Case descriptions, competencies/domains reflected upon
4. Looking back on action (self-assessment)	What went well? What were the challenges? What didn't go well?
5. Evidence considered	Feedback from assessment? Trainer feedback? Nurse feedback? Patient feedback? Unexpected outcomes of procedure? Own feelings?
6. Analysis	Describing why – for example, identifying cause and effect for unexpected case outcomes, or identifying reasons why progress is slow in one competency and fast in another
7. Formulating change	Identifying what actions you need to take to address any problems arising from reflection by adding items to the Personal Development Plan section of e-PDP

Reflection on tutorials

TABLE 5.7 Details of the reflections on tutorials

Number to be completed	The same number of tutorials conducted in practice (a minimum of 40)
Assessor	ES
How assessed	Each of the six sections within the e-PDP reflection response is reviewed and comments provided
Satisfactory performance	All six sections of the reflection response must be adequately completed, demonstrating active reflection

Table 5.8 outlines the six items that need to be completed for each reflection as prompted by e-PDP.

TABLE 5.8 Areas to be completed for the tutorial reflection

1. Date and Title	Confirming the date and subject of the tutorial
2. Length	The duration of the tutorial in hours (minimum of 1 hour)
3. Details	Case descriptions, competencies/domains reflected upon
4. Looking back on action (self-assessment)	What went well? What were the challenges? What didn't go well?
5. Analysis	Describing why – for example, identifying cause and effect for unexpected case outcomes, or identifying reasons why progress is slow in one competency and fast in another
6. Formulating change	Identifying what actions you need to take to address any problems arising from reflection by adding items to the PDP section of e-PDP

Reflection on study days

TABLE 5.9 Details of the study day reflections

Number to be completed	The same number of study days conducted throughout the year (usually 30)
Assessor	FTPD
How assessed	Each of the seven sections within the e-PDP reflection response is reviewed and comments provided
Satisfactory performance	All seven sections of the reflection response must be adequately completed, demonstrating active reflection

Table 5.10 outlines the six items that need to be completed for each reflection as prompted by e-PDP.

TABLE 5.10 Areas to be completed for the reflection on study days

1. Date and Title	Confirming the date and subject of the tutorial
2. Length	The duration of the study day in hours
3. Details	Case descriptions, competencies/domains reflected upon
4. Looking back on action (self-assessment)	What went well? What were the challenges? What didn't go well?
5. Evidence considered during reflection	Feedback from assessment? Trainer feedback? Nurse feedback? Patient feedback? Unexpected outcomes of procedure? Own feelings?
6. Analysis	Describing why – for example, identifying cause and effect for unexpected case outcomes, or identifying reasons why progress is slow in one competency and fast in another
7. Formulating change	Identifying what actions you need to take to address any problems arising from reflection by adding items to the PDP section of e-PDP

Patient survey (PAQ) reflection

TABLE 5.11 Details of the PAQ reflection

Number to be completed	Once during the year at Week 27
Assessor	ES and FTPD
How assessed	Each of the six sections within the e-PDP reflection response is reviewed and comments provided
Satisfactory performance	All six sections of the reflection response must be adequately completed, demonstrating active reflection

Table 5.12 outlines the seven items that need to be completed for the patient survey reflection as prompted by e-PDP.

TABLE 5.12 Areas to be completed for the PAQ reflection

1. Subject	Confirming the subject of the reflection
2. Date	Date relating to when you reflected upon the survey
3. Details	Method of the patient survey being collated
4. Looking back on action (self-assessment)	What went well? What were the challenges? What didn't go well?
5. Evidence considered	Feedback from assessment? Trainer feedback? Nurse feedback? Patient feedback? Unexpected outcomes of procedure? Own feelings?
6. Analysis	Describing why – for example, identifying cause and effect for unexpected case outcomes, or identifying reasons why progress is slow in one competency and fast in another
7. Formulating change	Identifying what actions you need to take to address any problems arising from reflection by adding items to the PDP section of e-PDP

FINAL APPRAISAL

This is a confidential part of your record of participation in FT and needs to be completed as a joint exercise by you and your ES.

TABLE 5.13 Details of the final appraisal

Number to be completed	One
Assessor	ES and FTPD
How assessed	Each of the five sections within the e-PDP reflection response, about your experience and achievements, is reviewed and comments provided
Satisfactory performance	All five sections of the reflection response must be adequately completed, demonstrating active reflection

Outlined here are the five areas that you would need to reflect on regarding your experience and achievements within the final appraisal section of e-PDP.
1. Patient care
2. Personal and professional development
3. Professional practice
4. Administration and management
5. Other comments

Usually conducted at Week 44 of the year, the FTPD must also complete a final summary informing the final decision for FT sign-off, documenting:
- how many study days you have attended
- whether you have completed a full training year
- whether you have completed the FT portfolio of evidence required
- whether you have completed the required number of assessments
- whether you have presented a key skill
- whether you have presented a case report
- whether you have presented a clinical audit
- whether you have completed your Dental Foundation Training e-Portfolio.

SCOTLAND

The assessments used within the e-Portfolio in Scotland are similar to the e-PDP, but they have been specifically designed for the practising arrangements in Scotland. Assessment is also different in that the e-Portfolio is submitted to a panel of assessors at the end of the training period. Unlike the rest of the UK, assessment also involves a summative test of knowledge, which informs the process of satisfactory completion.

The career
crossroads

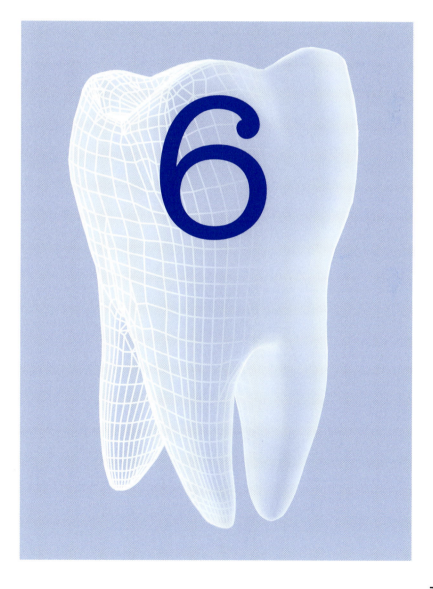

When you complete FT, you will have four main routes available to you, otherwise referred to as the career crossroads (*see* Figure 6.1).

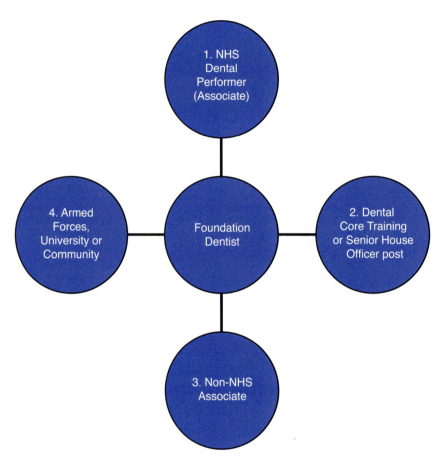

FIGURE 6.1 The career crossroads

1. NHS DENTAL PERFORMER (ASSOCIATE)

There are estimated to be 29 500 dentists practising in primary care settings in the UK, with the vast majority offering NHS dental treatment or a combination of NHS and private dental treatment.[83] UK dental practices are typically small or medium-sized businesses owned either by an individual or

---

83   Office of Fair Trading (OFT). *Dentistry: an OFT market study*. London: OFT; 2012.

a partnership of dentists, or they are owned by a corporate dental group (an incorporated company operating three or more dental practices).

The *British Dental Journal* is the usual place where positions are advertised, and it is common practice for you to apply by sending a covering letter or email and curriculum vitae (CV). Practice principals generally receive a high volume of applications for associate positions, so it is essential that your covering letter or email is catchy and your CV is concise. It is not a good idea to send pre-written references, as this is not considered authentic. Principals would rather request clinical references themselves, possibly using their own template.

Most FDs think that it will be hard for them to secure an associate role based on their quantitative clinical experience, but this is simply not true. Principals will also tend to look for the following features in a covering letter or email and CV:

- qualitative clinical experience
- interest in their practice/themselves
- written communication skills
- proximity to practice or realistic commute
- indication of career plan.

Covering letter or email

The purpose of a covering letter or email is to introduce your CV and to outline the reasons why you wish to apply for the advertised role at a particular practice; therefore, it should be personalised for each application. The covering letter or email should complement your CV, not repeat it, and should be no longer than a side of A4. If you are applying via email, take care not to send the same generic email to each practice.

CV

Limit your CV to two sides of A4 paper, typed in an easy-to-read font (such as 12-point Arial, Calibri, Georgia or Verdana) and subdivided into appropriate sections. If you are planning to email your CV, ensure that you save your CV as a .doc file, as some files cannot be readily opened by all computer software.

BOX 6.1 Template CV

Full name:

Professional details: GDC number, NHS performer number and defence organisation membership number

Personal details: contact details

Profile: this is your opportunity to use a few lines to showcase your qualities and professional interests

Education and qualifications: usually from undergraduate to postgraduate level, including any qualifications pending

Prizes and awards: received at university or during FT

Previous employment: starting with the most recent, including outside of dentistry; you should also provide an explanation of any gaps in your employment

Work experience: you could elaborate on what your duties are or were within each role

CPD: list the verifiable CPD courses attended relevant to the role applied for

Membership of professional bodies: such as the BDA and Faculty of General Dental Practice (FGDP)

Skills: these could include languages spoken, IT skills and driving licence

Interests: these could include your interests outside of dentistry including sport and music, but try to avoid documenting common interests such as socialising

Referees: the contact details of at least two clinical referees should be given

---

Interviews in general dental practice

Unlike dental school admissions and the FT national recruitment process, interviews in general dental practice are generally less formal. There is a wide range of approaches to the selection and interview process but it generally involves an interview with the practice owner or principal. The interviewer will generally want to glean from you whether you can demonstrate:

- a safe approach to caring for patients of the practice
- an attitude and ethos that fits in with the practice
- an awareness of the various operational constraints in general practice (such as equipment, materials and staffing)
- the capability of meeting an expected NHS or non-NHS target.

TABLE 6.1 Interview dos and don'ts

Do	Don't
Answer honestly, admitting when you don't know something	Pretend you know the answer to something, as you don't get points for attempting a question
Acknowledge any feedback, advising the interviewer how you intend to use that feedback	Be defensive or overly precious with your point of view
Be assertive with your answers	Come across as overconfident
Showcase any achievements that set you out from the crowd of applicants	Overstate your achievements
Ask questions to show your interest in the role	Focus your questions on financial matters
Be honest about your FT experiences	Offer irrelevant confidences
Remember that your interview usually begins as soon as you enter the practice and not necessarily when you are sitting opposite the interviewer	Be rude, short or abrupt to other members of the dental team

What's on offer?

If you apply for an NHS performer position at a practice it is likely that the provider, often the practice owner, will expect the performance of a set target of UDAs throughout the year. Commonly, full-time performers have contracts for 6000–7000 UDAs per annum, which allows some leeway for the provision of treatment on a private basis when the need arises. If we consider the notional target of 1875 UDAs expected of you as an FD, there is obviously a large gap between these figures, and you need to try to 'leap' this gap in the first year post FT.

While during FT you were employed by the practice owner and therefore protected by employment law, as an associate you will usually be regarded as a self-employed contractor. Employment law generally does not apply to an associate, and your relationship with the practice owner is governed by the specific terms of the contract you hold with them. This contract can be either verbal or written, but it is common for a provider–performer (or principal–associate) agreement to be formulated from the BDA template. Having a signed agreement protects both you and the provider and it should stipulate,

among other things, your annual UDA target. Whatever UDA target is nego-
tiated, it is important to review your performance regularly throughout the
year with the provider so that you can discuss the situation if you find that
your agreed UDA target proves to be beyond what you can ethically achieve
without dropping your standards. Other factors to consider when agreeing a
UDA target are whether you shall be taking over an established list of patients,
or whether there is an expectation to see new patients, and what the practice's
broken appointment (or 'failed to attend') rate is like. If expected to see new
patients to the practice, you cannot reasonably predict what their treatment
needs shall be and therefore how much of your time will be spent stabilising
oral disease as opposed to providing advanced restorations. Therefore, treating patients with higher treatment needs may mean that you need to work
harder to achieve a UDA target than you might expect.

 HINT! Aside from your annual UDA allocation, try to negotiate the following
points in your provider–performer agreement:
- the split of fees, laboratory bills and bad debts
- set number of holiday days per annum
- set number of days for study enabling you to comply with CPD
  requirements
- any requirement to use specific laboratories and materials
- with whom the responsibility lies for arranging and paying for locum
  cover in the event of sickness.

Temptation

It is easy to become lured by wishing to work in a desirable location, such
as in the bright lights of a city. Alongside this is the pressure of meeting the
fictional expectations of earning significantly more than you did during FT.
Whatever position you accept, beware of accepting it based on emotional or
financial drivers. By being financially driven you may find yourself placing
greater importance on meeting UDAs, or non-NHS financial targets, than on
the patient's needs, which may in turn risk compromising your clinical and
professional standards.

Corporate dentistry

In 2010, the corporate dental sector was estimated to account for around 10%
of the UK dentistry market.[84] With this share of the market expected to grow,

---

84   Laing & Buisson. *Dentistry UK Market Report*. London: Laing & Buisson; 2011. p. 8.

it is possible that you may be applying for an associate post within a practice operated by a corporate.

A natural progression from FT, where you have regular contact with your ES, is to work in a practice where the practice owner also works on-site. This situation in corporate practice is likely to be different as the clinical lead is frequently not on-site, which might not be helpful if you would prefer the safety net of a senior colleague closely supervising your progress. However, if you are confident to practise independently, then working in a practice with no on-site clinical lead should not be a concern – you could even become the clinical lead.

Corporates usually have robust systems and processes in place to ensure the delivery of financial profits, which can helpfully ensure that your UDA and private performance is target driven. However, compared with smaller practices you are likely to have less influence in how the practice is run, which may, for instance, affect your choice of dental materials to use. Although the face of a corporate in practice will usually be the practice manager, responsible for the practice's operational management, as a dentist you are still primarily responsible for ensuring that these standards are met in your surgery, or even across the entire practice.

 ACTION POINT! For most dentists, becoming an associate also means becoming self-employed. Remember to:
- register with HM Revenue and Customs (HMRC)
- pay Class 2 and 4 NI contributions
- open a business bank account
- save for future tax bills.

Practice ownership

Another option is to take the plunge into becoming a practice principal. FT will certainly help you to better understand practice management but you should be aware that running a practice involves a different skill set to performing dentistry. Before considering practice ownership you should access practice management advice and become aware of the marketplace. Being a principal involves being the 'accountable person' in the practice, not just because you become an employer but also because you may become the CQC registered provider and/or manager.

There is no blueprint defining practice ownership as being at the pinnacle of the career pathway for the general dental practitioner. In fact for many general dental practitioners being an associate often involves less responsibility than being a principal, also yielding greater financial return. That being said, practice ownership does have many attractions, such as managing people and setting your own working hours.

2. DENTAL CORE TRAINING OR SENIOR HOUSE OFFICER POST

Dental Core Training (DCT) posts are approved by Postgraduate Dental Deans for a maximum of 1 year and are available in hospital trusts, dental schools, the community dental services and general dental practice. The majority of these posts (DCT Year 1) are designed to follow on directly from the completion of FT. A smaller number of more senior posts (DCT Year 2 and DCT Year 3) will allow you to acquire additional skills in particular specialty areas after DCT Year 1, often as preparation for applying to join specialty training programmes. DCT posts were traditionally Senior House Officer posts, and some Senior House Officer posts still exist, such as in oral and maxillofacial surgery (OMFS). The recruitment process for DCT posts is not too dissimilar to the national recruitment process for FT.

Specialty training

All dentists at some point in their careers will probably have pondered whether they should enter a specialty or remain as a general practitioner. By specialising you will be restricting your scope of practice, at least for the short term; therefore, you must try to identify those aspects of dentistry that you are good at and which you find enjoyable. For instance, if you have always enjoyed treating children then you may wish to pursue this interest, as your passion for paediatric dentistry will see you through the training process. To test this passion it is vital that you obtain an insight into your chosen specialty by either shadowing or speaking with several specialists in the field. That way you will gain a further understanding of what the career entails and what you would be committing to.

You don't have to join a GDC Specialist List to practise any particular specialty, but you can only use the title 'specialist' if you are on the list. There are 13 specialist lists (OMFS is considered a specialty of medicine and not dentistry), with a brief description of each specialty[85] given in Table 6.2.

---

85   General Dental Council. Available at: www.gdcuk.org/Membersofpublic/Lookforaspecialist/Pages/
    default.aspx (accessed July 2013).

TABLE 6.2 GDC registrable specialties

Specialty	Description
Special care dentistry	Concerned with the improvement of the oral health of individuals and groups in society who have a physical, sensory, intellectual, mental, medical, emotional or social impairment or disability, or, more often, a combination of these factors; it pertains to adolescents and adults
Oral surgery	Deals with the treatment and ongoing management of irregularities and pathology of the jaw and mouth that require surgical intervention
Orthodontics	The development, prevention and correction of irregularities of the teeth, bite and jaw
Paediatric dentistry	Concerned with comprehensive therapeutic oral healthcare for children from birth through adolescence, including care for those who demonstrate intellectual, medical, physical, psychological and/or emotional problems
Endodontics	Concerned with the cause, diagnosis, prevention and treatment of diseases and injuries of the tooth root, dental pulp and surrounding tissue
Periodontics	The diagnosis, treatment and prevention of diseases and disorders (infections and inflammatory) of the gums and other structures around the teeth
Prosthodontics	The replacement of missing teeth and the associated soft and hard tissues by prostheses (crowns, bridges, dentures), which may be fixed or removable, or may be supported and retained by implants
Restorative dentistry	Deals with the restoration of diseased, injured, or abnormal teeth to normal function. Includes all aspects of endodontics, periodontics and prosthodontics
Dental public health	A non-clinical specialty involving the science and art of preventing oral diseases, promoting oral health to the population rather than the individual; it involves the assessment of dental health needs and ensuring dental services meet those needs
Oral medicine	Concerned with the oral healthcare of patients with chronic recurrent and medically related disorders of the mouth and with their diagnosis and non-surgical management
Oral microbiology	Diagnosis and assessment of facial infection – typically bacterial and fungal disease; this is a clinical specialty undertaken by laboratory-based personnel who provide reports and advice based on interpretation of microbiological samples
Oral and maxillofacial pathology	Diagnosis and assessment made from tissue changes characteristic of disease of the oral cavity, jaws and salivary glands; this is a clinical specialty undertaken by laboratory-based personnel
Dental and maxillofacial radiology	Involves all aspects of medical imaging that provide information about anatomy, function and diseased states of the teeth and jaws

Specialists are level 3 clinicians within the NHS national care pathways, and the journey towards specialising begins with completion of FT and DCT before going on to complete a specialty training programme. All dental specialty training programmes are of a minimum of 3 years' duration, with trainees referred to as specialty registrars (StRs). Following on from the national recruitment process for FT, in 2012 COPDEND trialed a similar process for NHS StR posts in England. The competition for specialty training programmes is brisk and it is favourable if you can demonstrate a wide range of experience through working in several specialist areas of dentistry. Master's degrees are an essential requirement for some specialties, with those available including:

- Master of Clinical Dentistry (MClinDent)
- Master of Science (MSc)
- Master of Dental Science (MDentSci)
- Master of Philosophy (MPhil).

Towards the end of the specialty training StRs sit the intercollegiate specialty fellowship examination and if successful, along with evidence of satisfactory completion of training provided by the LETB, will gain a Certificate of Completion of Specialty Training. The certificate will then allow the holder to be included on the GDC's specialist list for the chosen specialty. This then leads to eligibility to apply for NHS or academic/honorary consultant posts.

The Dental Gold Guide[86] is a guide for Postgraduate Dental Specialty Training produced by COPDEND following consultation with stakeholders and has the approval of the four UK health systems.

OMFS

OMFS is a surgical specialty concerned with the diagnosis and treatment of diseases affecting the mouth, jaws, face and neck. As OMFS has a dental and medical base, there exist various routes of entering a OMFS specialty training programme, which is usually of 5 years' duration. Completion of this programme leads to a Certificate of Completion of Training and being registered with the General Medical Council on the specialist list in oral and maxillofacial surgery, thereby becoming eligible for appointment as a consultant in oral and maxillofacial surgery within the NHS.

As an FD, to become eligible to apply for an OMFS specialty training programme you must first undertake a shortened medical course at a medical school before going on to complete core training in surgery.

---

86   COPDEND. *A Reference Guide for Postgraduate Dental Specialty Training in the UK: The Dental Gold Guide*. 3rd ed. 2013; Oxford: COPDEND.

Dentists with Enhanced Skills

DES, otherwise known as Dentists with Special Interests, are independent practitioners who provide services that are complementary to secondary care but within the primary care setting. DES are sort of a halfway house service between a primary care dental practitioner and a specialist; therefore, DES do not replace those services provided by a dentist who has undergone the training to gain entry onto the GDC specialist lists. DES are level 2 clinicians within the NHS national care pathways. The term 'DES' is not a protected title registrable with the GDC but rather an appointment or role given by NHS England when contracting with a DES to provide enhanced services to a local population.

For a dentist to work formally as a DES there is a process of accreditation by the employing or commissioning organisation, with the clinical competency frameworks providing a national system of assessment and evidence required to demonstrate competence for each special interest.[87]

3. NON-NHS ASSOCIATE

Non-NHS dentistry is commonly referred to as private dentistry, and there are dentists who carry out private dental treatment only,[88] but they constitute less than 10% of all dentists practising in primary care settings. Private dentistry accounts for approximately 42% of the UK dentistry market,[89] based on figures that do not include cosmetic dentistry. Non-NHS (private) dentistry generally comprises:

- *cosmetic dentistry* – primarily concerned with restoring or enhancing dental aesthetics
- *independent dentistry* – primarily concerned with rendering patients dentally fit on a fee-per-item basis
- *payment plan dentistry* – involves maintaining patients' dental fitness on a capitation basis.

Although the demand for private dentistry has recently softened,[90] this trend may change, as it is predicted that over the next few years the provision of NHS dental treatment may face increased pressure from cuts in public spending.[91]

---

87 Primary Care Contracting. *Dentists with Special Interests (DwSIs): a step by step guide to setting up a DwSI service.* London: NHS Primary Care Contracting; 2006.

88 Laing & Buisson. *Dentistry UK Market Report.* London: Laing & Buisson; 2011. p. 8.

89 Ibid. p. 4.

90 Ibid. p. 7.

91 Office of Fair Trading (OFT). *Dentistry: an OFT market study.* London: OFT; 2012.

4. THE ARMED FORCES, UNIVERSITY OR COMMUNITY

The defence dental services are a tri-service area employing approximately 1000 personnel from the three armed services and contracted civilians. Your role as a dentist would generally be to render armed service personnel dentally fit before being deployed on operational duty across the world. In the majority of cases, treatment is provided at service dental centres in the UK, but you may also have the opportunity to work abroad for short periods. Your career in the armed forces generally starts as a dental officer if you join having completed FT, or, alternatively, you could complete your FT in the defence dental services. If you do decide to join the armed forces you will need to undergo initial officer training, which may involve fitness development, military training and practical outdoor leadership challenges.

After FT you could apply to work as a clinical instructor to undergraduate dental students in a dental hospital, although this would generally be on a part-time basis. This role is usually a good starting point for a career as a clinical academic in a university. Although the criteria for promotion to a senior clinical academic position varies from one university to another, most require a PhD and an established research track record.

The community dental services (salaried dental services) enables you to work on a salaried basis in primary care community settings for patients who have difficulty accessing treatment in the general practice setting and who require additional services on a referral basis, such as domiciliary care. The community dental services are linked with the special care dentistry and paediatric specialties, and involve creating positive experiences for disadvantaged patients, including vulnerable adults and children. After FT you would typically start working as a dental officer caring for the full range of patients in a range of clinical settings, varying from community clinics to a patient's own home. There is also scope to progress your career as a senior dental officer offering care in a particular specialty and a clinical director, which is a clinical and management role.

PORTFOLIO CAREER

The choices that you make at the career crossroads are not irreversible and it is possible to head down one route before coming back to explore another route. Dentistry is often incredibly flexible and so it is even possible to travel down two routes at the same time; for instance, you could work part time as an NHS dental performer while also working part time as a clinical instructor in a dental hospital. Some individuals prefer this variety, building up a so-called portfolio career.

The four routes described earlier are not exhaustive and there are many other careers that you may wish to pursue – for instance, forensic dentistry or working in the dento-legal field. What is important is that you avoid looking at potential careers through rose-tinted glasses and instead gain some experience in your chosen field before embarking on the journey.

TAKING A CAREER BREAK

If after completing FT you are interested in taking a medium or long career break, you should ideally plan the break to understand what you need to do to enter clinical practice when you return. There are several areas that you would need to consider.

GDC registration

The GDC recommends that you should retain your UK registration when intending to take a break from dental work. If the 'break' is for less than a whole calendar year (January–December) then it will be more expensive to allow your registration with the GDC to lapse, as an additional restoration fee would be due. Whatever you decide, the CPD 'clock' will continue to tick. In other words, if you leave the Register and wish to restore in the future, you will be asked to show CPD, up to a maximum of 250 hours, in order to be able to restore.

NHS performer status

The NHS (Performers Lists) (England) Regulations 2013 outline that NHS England may remove a dental performer from the national dental performers list if they cannot demonstrate having performed dental services during the preceding 12 months.[92] This may mean applying for an NHS performers list assessment if you wish to return to primary care NHS dentistry, after having first found a practice that can offer you a position.

Refresher or retraining courses

When you return from a long break it is advisable to enrol onto a refresher or retraining hands-on course, which will enable you rebuild your confidence and regain your clinical procedural skills. If you do not have an active

---

92   The NHS (Performers Lists) (England) Regulations 2013, ¶14 (5).

NHS performer number then it is likely that you may be charged by a post-graduate dental centre if you wish to enrol onto a Section 63 or otherwise NHS-funded course. It is also advisable to produce a personal development plan, enabling you to plan your return to work with a suitable mentor from Health Education England.

MFDS AND MJDF

There are two initial postgraduate qualifications available to you:
1. the Diploma of Membership of the Joint Dental Faculties of the Royal College of Surgeons of England (MJDF RCS Eng)
2. the Diploma of Membership of the Faculty of Dental Surgery of either the Royal College of Surgeons of Edinburgh (MFDS RCS Ed) or the Royal College of Physicians and Surgeons of Glasgow (MFDS RCPS Glas).

The end point of the Dental Foundation Programme is achieved by the demonstration of competencies over the prescribed one year period, and it does not require the achievement of the MFDS or MJDF qualification.[93] Nevertheless many regard the MFDS or MJDF qualifications as marking the informal end point of FT and Dental Core Training Year 1. With the MFDS and MJDF syllabi clearly aligned to the COPDEND Dental Foundation Training Curriculum, your FT experience will naturally assist in your preparation for the requisite examinations.

The format and cost of examinations for the MFDS and MJDF qualifications are broadly similar, with an annual subscription payable to the college in which you have taken the exams in order to use the post-nominal letters. Annual subscription also offers a range of benefits specific to that college.

There also exists the Diploma of Membership of the Faculty of Dentistry Royal College of Surgeons in Ireland (MFD RCSI).

There is no specific advantage in gaining one qualification over another, since they all offer benefits from the primary and secondary care perspective. FDs sit the MFDS, MJDF or MFD examinations for a variety of reasons, such as enhancing job prospects, gaining post-nominal letters and career development. Obtaining the MFDS, MJDF or MFD has traditionally served as an entry requirement for specialist training. However, this changed when the GDC agreed that there will be no formal examination entry requirement, with selection more likely to be on the basis of a range of criteria demonstrating

---

93   COPDEND. *Dental Foundation Training Policy Statement*, ¶38. Available at: www.copdend.org/content.aspx?Group=foundation&Page=foundation_policystatement (accessed November 2013).

suitability. Therefore, although possession of a postgraduate qualification such as the MFDS, MJDF or Membership of the Faculty of Dentistry (MFD) diploma is not essential, it is desirable for entry into specialty training.

The eligibility criteria for sitting Part 1 examination of both the MJDF and MFDS include being in possession of a recognised primary dental qualification, but there is no specified time requirement of working in clinical practice. Therefore, you can sit Part 1 during your FT year, which would make sense, as the syllabus for both the MFDS and the MJDF examinations are aligned to the COPDEND Dental Foundation Training Curriculum.

 TIP! Part 1 examinations for MFDS and MJDF are held twice a year, in October and April. Some FDs would rather complete the examination during FT in October in order to best utilise the knowledge acquired at undergraduate level. Please be aware that October might be too soon to prepare for a professional examination, as this is a critical stage of your FT year when you will still be 'finding your way' in practice.

GETTING INVOLVED

One of the rewarding aspects of FT is knowing that you are not alone in experiencing the ups and downs of clinical practice. The peer learning and support gained from other FDs within your scheme is key towards helping you deal with all sorts of challenges. Depending upon your chosen career pathway after FT, however, the opportunity for peer support generally wanes. It is important not to remain secluded from your peers but, rather, to get involved in the various established professional networks and committees that exist:

- Dental local professional networks (LPNs)
- LDCs
- BDA branch sections
- FGDP divisions.

Dental LPNs aim to be considered as the 'authentic clinical voice' for the local dental profession. They are a non-political network typically comprising a clinical chair, patient representative, specialists such as a consultant in dental public health, NHS England and local clinicians from across the clinical spectrum[94] (primary care, secondary care and the salaried dental care services and possibly the non-NHS sector). Among their other functions, dental LPNs

---

94   NHS England. *Local Professional Networks: single operating framework*. London: NHS England; 2013.

work closely with the NHS England Area Team to provide clinical input in the commissioning of primary care, to deliver and develop cohesive oral health strategies and to drive quality improvement.

You must be a BDA member to be involved in local BDA branch section meetings and likewise must be a member of the FGDP to be involved in divisional meetings; the only stipulation to being involved with your LDC is that you contribute to the statutory levy as an NHS dental performer. LDCs are statutory bodies representing the interests of local NHS GDPs (both performers and providers) with the discretion to also represent dentists working in the local salaried services. LDCs are influential within the dental profession, acting as a strong source of advice to GDPs and traditionally acting as a sounding board to local NHS commissioning decisions. Some LDCs also manage Practitioner Advice and Support Scheme groups, which act as a resource for GDPs with health-, conduct- and performance-related issues.

FUTURE-PROOFING

Changes to the demography of the UK include the number of people over 85 being projected to increase from 1.4 million in 2010 to 1.9 million by 2020 and to 3.5 million by 2035.[95] As older patients are retaining their natural teeth for longer, a population with a higher number of older people will have complex treatment needs that will need to be met by dental care provided in a range of different settings, such as in residential homes and patients' own homes. The treatment of older people with more complex needs also involves issues in gaining valid consent and determining appropriate treatment for those entering their end of life. One part of future-proofing your service skills would be to gain experience in gerodontology and the provision of domiciliary dental care.

---

95 Office for National Statistics. *News Release: UK population projected to hit 70m by 2027.* Office for National Statistics; 2011.

Dento-legal considerations

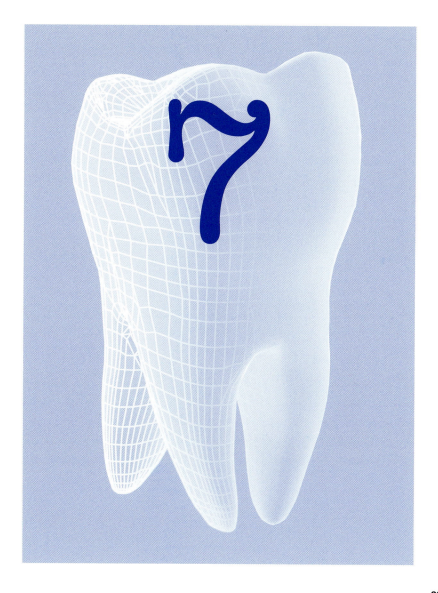

You are engaged on the understanding that you are skilled to perform certain duties and will do so with reasonable care. Although your ES and/or practice owner as your employer takes full responsibility under their contract with NHS England for your acts and omissions (through vicarious liability), this does not divorce you from needing to comply with your obligations as:

- a dental performer under the NHS (Performers Lists) (England) Regulations 2013, and
- a GDC registrant.

Indeed, as an FD you could appear before the GDC as a fully registered practitioner, in your own right, to investigate your fitness to practise by reason of your:

- conduct, including convictions and cautions (if you fall short of the code of conduct laid down in the GDC's *Standards for the Dental Team*)
- performance (if you fall short of the various clinical standards), or
- health.

 READING POINT! You can access the GDC's *Standards for the Dental Team* at: www.gdc-uk.org/Dentalprofessionals/Standards/Documents/Standards%20 for%20the%20Dental%20Team.pdf

 READING POINT! You can read about the specific charges, findings of fact and determinations found against registrants by GDC committee members from the hearings section of the GDC website at: www.gdc-uk.org/Membersofpublic/ Hearings/Pages/Hearings-list.aspx

EMPLOYMENT LAW

You will be employed by either your ES, or the practice owner, whose obligations towards you and other employed staff at the practice will already exist. These include obligations under the Health and Safety at Work etc. Act 1974. Your Foundation Contract complies with the Employment Rights Act 1996 (as amended) (Contracts of Employment and Redundancy Payments Act (Northern Ireland) 1965 as amended).

CPD

The GDC introduced continuing professional development (CPD) for dentists in 2002, which you need to participate in by law. The GDC has defined CPD as:

> lectures, seminars, courses, individual study and other activities, that can be included in your CPD record if it can be reasonably expected to advance your professional development as a dentist or dental care professional and is relevant to your practice or intended practice.[96]

'Verifiable' CPD must meet specific conditions, whereas 'general' CPD is educational activities that are not independently verified, such as private study. Dentists must carry out at least 250 hours of CPD every 5 years in a CPD cycle, with at least 75 of these hours needing to be verifiable. Although this theoretically could mean that you could spend just 1 year of every 5 'clocking up' your CPD requirements, it is recommended that your attendance is spaced out across your CPD cycle. The GDC expects dentists to complete the following three core subjects of CPD:[97]

1. Medical emergencies – 10 hours per CPD cycle (works out to 2 hours each year)
2. Disinfection and decontamination – 5 hours per CPD cycle (works out to 1 hour each year)
3. Radiography and radiation protection – 5 hours per CPD cycle (works out to 1 hour each year).

Also, the GDC recommends accessing CPD in the following areas:
- Legal and ethical issues
- Complaints handling
- Oral cancer early detection.

An understanding of the importance of CPD within dentistry and its recording is a COPDEND curriculum competency[98] that you are expected to demonstrate during FT. As an FD your first CPD cycle will not commence at the point of GDC registration, but rather at the beginning of the first full calendar year following registration, i.e. from 1 January. This means that any CPD you

---

96 General Dental Council. *Continuing Professional Development for Dental Professionals.* London: General Dental Council; 2013. p. 5.
97 Ibid., pp. 14 and 15.
98 Committee of Postgraduate Dental Deans and Directors UK (COPDEND). *Interim Dental Foundation Training Curriculum & Assessment Framework Guidance 2013–2014.* Oxford: COPDEND; 2013 professionalism domain, ¶3 (3).

accrue in the period between the point of registration and 31 December of that calendar year will not count towards your CPD cycle. During FT you will cover a minimum of 30 study days which, if verifiable, may mean that you could complete close to the full 75 hours expected of you within the first calendar year of your CPD cycle. This could affect your desire to complete any other verifiable CPD activities during the remainder of that CPD cycle. Therefore, it is common for your FTPD to issue you with a verifiable CPD certificate for a fixed number of hours (i.e. 25 hours) upon completion of the FT programme, which can contribute towards your CPD cycle. Of course, any verifiable CPD activities completed outside of FT in the first calendar year following registration will count towards your CPD cycle.

You must keep a record of all the CPD hours that you do, both verifiable (for which you must also keep documentary proof from the activity provider) and general. This is because every year you will be required to submit to the GDC the number of verifiable and general CPD hours completed, which can be done either online at www.eGDC-uk.org or by completing an annual declaration form. Although evidence of CPD may be requested, GDC registrants currently enjoy the privilege of self-regulation, which is accompanied by a responsibility of maintaining the highest standards of ethical practice. However, the GDC is working to introduce a system of revalidation,[99] which is already mandatory for doctors. Revalidation is the process by which individuals are required to demonstrate on a regular basis that they are up to date and fit to practise.

COMPLAINTS

As a dental student you are generally sheltered from complaints and litigation, as you tend to treat patients generally at no cost, within highly supervised clinics. The culture in general dental practice, however, is different, as patients pay NHS charges, or the state does on their behalf, which acts to increase their expectations of the standard of care provided. Patients are empowered to give feedback on their dental experiences, and are quick to say when they are dissatisfied with their experience. In this regard dental practices are no different from restaurants and hotels in being reviewed and scrutinised, increasingly online. The reality is that we live in a less forgiving and more litigious climate, and this can be a scary prospect.

A complaint is generally regarded to be any expression of dissatisfaction

---

99   GDC. Available at: www.gdc-uk.org/Aboutus/policy/Pages/policyitem.aspx?AspXPage=g_382DFC4 7F60D4C7FA30F9851641648E4:%2540Title%3DRevalidation (accessed November 2013).

with a service that you have provided to a patient. The GDC expect you to normally respond to a complaint in writing or by phone as soon as you receive it, if possible. If you cannot sort the complaint out immediately, you should normally send an acknowledgement within 3 working days of receiving the complaint and respond to the complaint no later than 10 working days after receiving it. This may be different, however, if there are exceptional circumstances or if you have agreed a different timescale with the patient.[100] All written responses to NHS complaints need to be counter-signed by the Responsible Person in the practice who is usually the practice owner. If a complaint cannot be resolved locally then patients have recourse to the *Dental Complaints Service* regarding private treatment and the *Parliamentary and Health Service Ombudsman* regarding NHS services, where the NHS contract provider is likely to be questioned. Please note however that the Foundation Contract obliges you to comply with the NHS Terms of Service.

A 2012 survey conducted by Cardiff University revealed that 11% of the 510 trainers who responded indicated experiencing difficulties related to patient complaints about their trainee's work or attitude.[101] Receiving a complaint does not necessarily mean that you are a 'bad dentist' as there are many reasons why a patient would feel the need to complain. However, one of the main reasons why dentists are sued is because the patient's questions are not answered.[102] Evidence also supports the fact that good communication skills are key towards ensuring that patients remain satisfied regardless of the quality of care they receive.[103] Patients who feel informed and involved in deciding the most appropriate treatment for their condition are more likely to comply with it and less likely to complain when things go wrong.

Research suggests that there are two sets of factors that influence patients' decision to sue or seek redress:
1. *predisposing factors* – rudeness, delays, inattentiveness, miscommunication, apathy, no communication
2. *precipitating factors* – adverse outcomes, iatrogenic injury, failure to provide adequate care, mistakes, incorrect care, systems errors.[104]

100 GDC. *Principles of Complaints Handling.* London: GDC; 2009, standard 4.4.
101 Gilmour A, Jones R, Bullock AD. *Dental Foundation Trainers' Expectations of a Dental Graduate.* Final Report. Cardiff: Wales Deanery/Cardiff University; 2012. p. 14.
102 Krause HR, Bremerich A, Rustemeyer J. Reasons for patients' discontent and litigation. *J Craniomaxillofac Surg.* 2001; **29**(3): 181–3.
103 DiMatteo MR, Hays RD, Prince LM. Relationship of physicians' nonverbal communication skill to patient satisfaction, appointment noncompliance, and physician workload. *Health Psychol.* 1986; **5**(6): 581–94.
104 Bunting RF Jr, Benton J, Morgan WD. Practical risk management principles for physicians. *J Healthc Risk Manag.* 1998; **18**(4): 29–53.

Precipitating factors on their own are unlikely to lead to litigation in the absence of the predisposing factors that build up a patient's dissatisfaction over time. These predisposing factors can manifest through patient groans and gripes. If you identify these groans or gripes then you should act to respond to these promptly and in an empathetic manner before they have the opportunity to grow into formal complaints. In fact listening effectively and being responsive to non-verbal cues is a COPDEND curriculum competency[105] that you are expected to demonstrate during FT. Your attitude to patient complaints should be proactive rather than reactive with your default position being to ask members of your dental team at the end of the day whether any patients made groans or gripes that you could help to resolve.

Having a professional approach to patients' complaints and accepting responsibility for your actions where appropriate is a COPDEND curriculum competency[106] that you are expected to demonstrate during FT. If you receive a complaint, whether written or verbal, you would need to highlight this to your ES. All complaints should be acknowledged quickly, informing the patient when they may receive a formal response. There is then the opportunity to investigate the complaint, identifying all members of the dental team involved and seeking their views before a formal response is drafted. It is at this stage that you may wish to contact your defence organisation. The response should be sympathetic and aim to resolve the patient's dissatisfaction. Following up the complaint is important, as is reflecting upon the matter.

 TIP! 'Sorry' should not be the hardest word when responding to a complaint. Apologising when something has not gone according to plan is not an admission of liability; therefore, you can be sorry for the dissatisfaction caused. Often that is all that the patient wants to hear.

Trust and goodwill underpin the dentist–patient relationship. Patients have a right to trust their dentist, and as standard 1.3.1 of the GDC's *Standards for the Dental Team*[107] stipulates:

> You must justify the trust that patients, the public and your colleagues place in you by always acting honestly and fairly in your dealings with them.

---

105 Committee of Postgraduate Dental Deans and Directors UK (COPDEND). *Interim Dental Foundation Training Curriculum & Assessment Framework Guidance 2013–2014*. Oxford: COPDEND; 2013 communication domain, ¶1 (11).

106 Ibid.; 2013 professionalism domain, ¶1 (3).

107 General Dental Council. *Standards for the Dental Team*. London: General Dental Council; 2013.

Research has shown that twice as many people in the UK trust their dentist as their family doctor,[108] which sets a strong precedent for you to follow with your patients. This is clearly important, as more than 75% of those surveyed also claimed to follow their dentist's advice in terms of frequency of visits.

Goodwill is the intangible asset that represents good customer relations and is part of what makes a patient visit you at your practice, and not another. Being friendly and empathetic with your patients helps to build layers of goodwill that can insulate you from potential complaints when the outcome of treatment does not go according to plan. This is where the old adage 'never treat a stranger' applies, which incidentally is the best insurance against dissatisfied patients.

> *Be nicer than necessary to everyone you meet. Everyone is fighting some kind of battle.*
>
> —Socrates (470–399 BC)

A common mistake of the FD is to treat patients as if working on a phantom head. We must not forget the service element of dentistry, as it will be the people, not the teeth, who will complain if dissatisfied. Effective communication is key, as asserted by Yamalik[109] who identifies the need for dentists to avoid technical language and patronising behaviour. Patients will want to hear about the benefits to them of dental treatment, and not just about the dentistry itself. The use of more basic language as opposed to more technical terms can even be found to reduce anxiety prior to treatment.[110]

RECOVERING FROM COMPLAINTS

It is hard not to take complaints personally; after all, complaints are expressions of dissatisfaction. Furthermore as a dentist there is no faceless organisation to hide behind as there is only you who must 'face the music'. After a complaint has been resolved, there are commonly two approaches taken:
1. To rationalise the ordeal as a 'bad day at the office' before carrying on myopically, or

---

108 British Dental Trade Association. *Perceptions of Dentistry and Motivation Research*. Chesham: British Dental Trade Association; Online poll of 5589 UK respondents aged between 18 and 55; April 2012.

109 Yamalik N. Dentist-patient relationship and quality care 3. Communication. *Int Dent J*. 2005; **55**(4): 254–6.

110 Lipp M, Dick W, Daubländer M, *et al.* [Different information patterns and their influence on patient anxiety before dental local anaesthesia] [German]. *Dtsch Z Mund Kiefer Gesichtschir*. 1991; **15**(6): 449–57.

2. To reflect on the experience, conceding any weaknesses before thinking about how you can learn from them.

The second approach is generally considered to be the more successful in preventing the same type of complaint from recurring. However, both approaches can result in you losing confidence particularly with the delivery of comparable future care. This can in turn affect your competence if you allow it to. It is so important to seek impartial feedback from somebody when reflecting on a complaint because it is only natural for us to be slightly subjective and overgenerous with the critique of our own performance. This feedback could be sought from your FTPD or defence organisation. A complaint should not be regarded as a 'negative' but more of a performance improvement indicator. Reflecting should allow you to identify your specific skills, clinical or other, which contributed to the predisposing and precipitating factors of the complaint. Then just as with performing any other skill, such as riding a bicycle, the correction of the identified skills needs to occur responsively so as to not affect your future performance, just as you would correct handlebar over-steer to retain your balance on the bicycle.

ATTITUDE

Many consider knowledge, skills and attitudes to be the fundamental building blocks of all effective training, including FT. While your skills are underpinned by knowledge, with the ability to improve them through deliberate practice, attitudes are also important to develop. Attitudes are the established ways of responding to people and situations, based on the beliefs, values and assumptions that we hold. How we respond to situations, and our behaviour, can reflect our attitude.

Attitude is so important in healthcare that a study conducted in the United States[111] found that differences in the attitudes and behaviours of doctors can determine those who had never been sued and those who had been sued frequently. The most significant differentiating feature between these different groups was not the actual treatment provided, but the way in which it was delivered. The study found that the perceived characteristics of doctors who were most likely to be sued were:
● an unwillingness to listen

---

111 Hickson GB, Clayton EW, Entman SS, *et al.* Obstetricians' prior malpractice experience and patients' satisfaction with care. *JAMA.* 1994; **272**(20): 1583–7.

- an appearance of not having sufficient time for their patients, or of being rushed
- an impression of disinterest or even arrogance
- perceived lack of care and concern.

Alongside your clinical skills, your reputation is one of the most valuable professional assets that you shall have during your FT year. However, unlike clinical skills, your reputation can be lost very quickly and this can be due to your attitude.

> *Your attitude, not your aptitude, will determine your altitude.*
>
> —Zig Ziglar (1926–2012)

COMMUNICATING EXPECTATIONS

Often patients will present with a clear idea of what treatment outcome they are expecting, which may sometimes be unrealistic. As patients are not identical, if patients have based their expectations on an outcome achieved for another patient, it is important to communicate why their particular case may prevent the same outcome being reached.

The patient's perception of clinically successful treatment differs to that of the dentist. Therefore, it is very possible that a treatment performed competently and non-negligently may have a complaint attached to it if there is an inadequate understanding of the patient's expectations from the outset, followed up with effective communication. Effective communication involves not only conveying information to the patient but also attentively listening to them.

It is best to understand patient expectations from the outset and then to understand where these expectations arise from by spending time with each patient. That way it will be easier to keep them in touch with realistic results, and a sure fire way of not making promises that you will not be able to keep.

You must also bear in mind that different generational expectations exist. *Generational theory*, as originally promoted by Neil Howe and William Strauss,[112] suggests that there are value bases to each generation that have been shaped during our formative years and influenced by social, political, economic and cultural events with a global reach. As an FD it is likely that

---

112 Howe N, Strauss W. *Generations: the history of America's future, 1584 to 2069*. Reprint edition. New York: Perennial; 1992.

you belong to *Generation Y* (born between 1990 and the present), and will need to care for patients belonging to the older *veterans* (born between 1929 and 1945), *baby boomers* (born between 1946 and 1967) and *Generation X* (born between 1968 and 1989). This could create communication challenges as older generations may hold differing priorities, preferring to use a different vocabulary while interpreting phrases differently to you. For instance, as a Generation Y you may want to explain how a procedure is performed utilising the best technology, but a baby boomer may just want to understand the outcomes of treatment. You should try to bear in mind these differences before tailoring your communication to your patients, thereby ensuring that you meet their expectations.

 TIP! It is common, when first starting out, for patients to comment on you being 'too young to be a dentist'.

> One way of responding is to outline how long it has taken you to become a practising dentist and that you have had the privilege of being taught the latest skills and techniques. If you respond in a confident manner then patients are more likely to develop confidence in your competence.

NEGLIGENCE

While the *Oxford English Dictionary*'s definition of negligence[113] is a *'failure to take proper care over something'*, in fact, for a dentist to be successfully sued for negligence there are three questions that would need to be addressed, otherwise referred to as the 'negligence equation':

1. Was a duty of care owed to the patient? Usually this answer is yes, by the nature of the established duty between dentist and patient.
2. Had the duty of care been breached? This involves setting the professional standard of care expected by the patient and then applying that standard to the dentist's actions or omissions.
3. Did an injury or damage result from the breach? This involves demonstrating that the breach of duty was the factual cause of the damage.

As was demonstrated in the case *Wilsher v Essex Area Health Authority* [1987] QB 730, inexperience is not considered as a tool to lower the required professional standard of care delivered to a patient. Therefore, as an FD the standard of care that you will be expected to deliver will be the same as that of

---

113 Oxford English Dictionary. Available at: www.oxforddictionaries.com/ (accessed November 2013).

a reasonably competent practitioner within the same field. Although this may be considered as unfair, you must consider that a patient is entitled to expect a duty of care that relates not to the individual but to the post that the health-care professional occupies, which in this case is a dental performer. So, who is responsible in the case of a claim arising against you? You, your ES, the LETB, or all three? There is no simple answer to this question since it all depends upon the intricacies of each individual case. But generally speaking, whereas the LETB is responsible for overseeing your training, and your employer (your ES or practice owner) remains vicariously liable for your actions or omissions, you would still be expected to answer to claims made about some aspects of your treatment. This is why it is vital that you successfully indemnify yourself by taking out professional indemnity cover from a dental defence organisa-tion. Where you have co-treated or treatment-planned a patient with your ES, the responsibility to respond to a claim would be shared, and if that claim were to be successful then liability may need to be apportioned.

GUIDELINES

A guideline is considered to be a statement by which to determine a course of action, and clinical guidelines are published by a number of bodies, includ-ing NICE, who act to:[114]

> provide independent, authoritative and evidence-based guidance on the most effective ways to prevent, diagnose and treat disease and ill health, reducing inequalities and variation.

There are some who feel that guidelines give rise to the practice of 'cookbook dentistry', whereby dentists are at risk of practising prescriptively, even when it may be justified to use clinical discretion in the patient's best interests. The judiciary, however, has held professional guidelines as the legal standard in which to find negligence, such as in the case of *JAC Richards v Swansea NHS Trust* [2007] EWHC 487 (QB). Therefore, it is important to recognise and fol-low guidelines.

---

114 Available at: www.nice.org.uk/aboutnice/ (accessed November 2013).

ACTION POINT! Here are some clinical guidelines applicable to general dental practice. Can you think of any others?
- NICE guidance on the extraction of wisdom teeth*
- FGDP (UK) *Adult Antimicrobial Prescribing in Primary Dental Care for GDPs*†
- ....
- ....

* NICE Technology Appraisal Guidance – No.1. *Guidance on the Extraction of Wisdom Teeth*; March 2000.
† FGDP (UK). *Adult Antimicrobial Prescribing in Primary Dental Care for GDPs.* 2nd ed. London: FGDP (UK); 2012.

CQC

The Health and Social Care Act 2008 established a single health and social care regulator in England, the Care Quality Commission (CQC). The CQC has a responsibility to ensure that all health and social care services in England provide people with safe, effective, compassionate and high-quality care. For dentistry this includes hospitals and all dental practices.

The CQC carries out its functions through inspecting all services against the same standards of safety and quality. The CQC's definitions of the five questions that they ask about quality and safety are whether the service (1) safe, (2) effective, (3) caring, (4) responsive and (5) well led. This is set out into six different sections,[115] each with outcomes not all of which will be applicable to dentistry:

1. involvement and information
2. personalised care, treatment and support
3. safeguarding and safety
4. suitability of staffing
5. quality and management
6. suitability of management.

There is a Memorandum of Understanding between the CQC and the GDC that sees the two regulators share information about dental services, thereby promoting patient safety.

---

115 Care Quality Commission. *Guidance about Compliance: essential standards of quality and safety.* London: Care Quality Commission; 2010.

CLINICAL GOVERNANCE

To comply with legislative, contractual and regulatory requirements, your practice will more than likely evidence compliance with clinical governance requirements through the maintenance of a clinical governance (or CQC outcomes) folder. Clinical governance has been defined as:

> A framework through which NHS organisations are accountable for continuously improving the quality of their services and safeguarding high standards of care by creating an environment in which excellence in clinical care will flourish.[116]

Therefore, clinical governance is essentially a quality assurance process involving the steps and procedures taken to ensure that patients encounter a high quality of care. Quality has been found to include the following aspects:

- patient safety
- patient experience
- effectiveness of care.[117]

Quality care is not achieved by focusing on one or two aspects of this definition; high-quality care encompasses all three aspects with equal importance being placed on each. Quality, however, is a moving target; therefore, it is important that a practice's clinical governance requirements be continuously reviewed. The *Primary Care Dental Services: Clinical Governance Framework*[118] is based on the Department of Health's publication *Standards for Better Health*[119] and outlines the following 12 themes:

1. Infection Control
2. Child Protection
3. Dental Radiography
4. Staff, Patient & Public Safety
5. Evidence Based Practice & Research
6. Prevention & Public Health
7. Clinical Records, Patient Privacy, Confidentiality
8. Support Staff Involvement & Development
9. Clinical Team Requirements & Development

---

116 Department of Health. *A First Class Service: quality in the new NHS*. London: Department of Health; 1998.

117 Darzi A. Quality and the NHS Next Stage Review. *Lancet*. 2008; **371**(9624): 1563–4.

118 Primary Care Contracting. *Primary Care Dental Services: clinical governance framework*. London: Primary Care Contracting; 2006.

119 Department of Health. *Standards for Better Health*. London: Department of Health; 2004.

10. Patient Information & Involvement
11. Fair & Accessible Care
12. Clinical Audit & Peer Review.

RECORDS

Clinical records permit a patient's care and treatment to be documented for future access by healthcare professionals, the patient and a number of bodies who may have a legal right of access. Where there is a conflict of evidence between a dentist's and patient's version of events, the patient's version is usually preferred unless the records can provide clear evidence to support the dentist's account. Reciting the care and treatment provided from memory is susceptible to bias and misattribution; therefore, keeping proper clinical records is arguably your strongest defence in a complaint or negligence claim. Always remember:

> If it's not written down, then it didn't happen.

Although you may be familiar with writing generous amounts of clinical record entries at dental school, this is usually known to change in general practice, either because of time constraints or because of access to IT software templates, abbreviations and/or codes. Your clinical record entries need to be able to capture your encounter with patients, and therefore need to be crystal clear, comprehensive and contemporaneous. The full, accurate and secure maintenance of patients' records is a COPDEND curriculum competency[120] that you are expected to demonstrate during FT.

Keeping proper records of the care and treatment that you provide forms an essential part of your overall duty of care. It is not only a GDC and CQC requirement but also an NHS contractual one, as outlined in part 13, clause 202, of the General Dental Services Contract:

> The Contractor shall ensure that a full, accurate and contemporaneous record is kept in the patient record in respect of the care and treatment given to each patient under the Contract, including treatment given to a patient who is referred to the Contractor.

---

120 Committee of Postgraduate Dental Deans and Directors UK (COPDEND). *Interim Dental Foundation Training Curriculum & Assessment Framework Guidance 2013–2014*. Oxford: COPDEND; 2013. Management and leadership domain, ¶1 (4).

TABLE 7.1 Record-keeping structure

Process	What to record
1. History	• Reason for attendance • Symptoms • Previous dental history • Social history • Oral hygiene habits • Personal wishes/expectations
2. Examination	Charting of the dentition, Basic Periodontal Examination for patients from around the age of 13, extra-oral and intra-oral soft tissue negative as well as positive findings (such as 'no swelling')
3. Discussion with patient	The information relayed to the patient about your findings resulting from history and examination, together with his or her responses
4. Special investigations	The justification and evaluation of all special investigations conducted; for radiographs this would also include documenting quality ratings
5. Diagnoses and prognoses	The identification of the nature of disorders or diseases processes along with a forecast of their development
6. Treatment plan	Details of the sequenced treatment to be provided within that course of treatment FP17DC must be completed for all Band 2 and 3 treatments* or where private treatment is also proposed
7. Consent (and specific warnings)	The information relayed to the patient regarding the treatment proposal including procedures, risks, benefits, alternatives, costs and the condition of the patient; it also includes any questions asked, along with your responses
8. Treatment provided (including disease stabilisation and any advanced treatment)	Advice on oral hygiene and general health. Details of the procedures performed, the anatomical structures involved, all materials used and drugs administered (including type, route, dosage, frequency and quantity); it also includes the outcome of treatment. Details of pre- and postoperative instructions given should also be recorded
9. Recall	The oral disease risk level (high, medium or low) assigned to the patient along with a prescribed recall interval in months ranging from 3 to 24 months[†]

* The NHS (General Dental Services Contracts) Regulations 2005 P6 S3 P2, ¶7 (5).

[†] NICE Clinical Guideline 19. *Dental Recall: recall interval between routine dental examinations*; October 2004.

Your records should be methodical and document a stepwise approach to patient assessment and treatment,[121] also showing evidence of the thought processes behind the decisions made. Table 7.1 outlines a generic structure of what to record, which is not exhaustive.

Be careful not to write any inappropriate comments about a patient, or their condition, in the clinical records since the patient has access to the records. This could cause irreversible damage to the trusting relationship that you hold with them.

Particularly with electronic records, there can be instances when a part of the clinical records becomes unavailable, due to computer malfunction, when a patient attends for treatment. Under these circumstances do not be forced into blindly treating the patient. You should inform the patient and decide whether to go ahead with the appointment without access to past clinical information. Sometimes it is safer to reschedule the appointment.

> **BEWARE!** It can be tempting to revisit and amend clinical record entries after the event, especially in light of a complaint or claim being received. Performing such an act is looked upon very unfavourably by the GDC, who consider this to be a dishonest act, risking a severe sanction.

CONSENT

The word 'autonomy' is taken from the Greek for self-determination, and for Beauchamp and Childress[122] respect for autonomy is one of four equal principles of biomedical ethics which essentially holds that a person's right to decide how to live their life is respected. Gillon[123] asserts that autonomy is regarded as the *'first among equals'* and is seen as a rejection of paternalism, where the dentist decides what is important for the patient. Respect for autonomy is central to the concept of 'informed consent' which is a familiar and ethically important aspect of everyday transactions such as shopping for groceries or borrowing a book from the library. But this is only ethically acceptable if all parties to the transaction take part willingly in awareness of ways in which others' proposed actions will bear on them.[124]

121 FGDP (UK). *Clinical Examination and Record-Keeping: good practice guidelines*. 2nd ed. FGDP(UK)'s series of standards for dental professionals; 2009.

122 Beauchamp TL, Childress JF. *Principles of Biomedical Ethics*. 4th ed. Oxford University Press; 1994.

123 Gillon R. Ethics needs principles – four can encompass the rest – and respect for autonomy should be 'first among equals'. *J Med Ethics*. 2003; **29**: 307–12.

124 O'Neill O. Some limits of informed consent. *J Med Ethics*. 2003; **29**: 4–7.

If there was any doubt regarding the importance that the courts place on patient autonomy at the expense of paternalism in medical law, this was eliminated in *Chester v Afshar [2004]* UKHL 41. This case was heard not long after the entry into force of the Human Rights Act 2000 during an era within which judges paid more attention to the patient's rights such as Article 8 in the European Convention on Human Rights, the right to respect for private and family life. In *Chester v Afshar [2004]* UKHL 41, despite a surgical procedure being performed non-negligently by Mr Afshar and despite an entirely foreseeable risk not being found to be a direct cause of injury, Mr Afshar's failure to warn Ms Chester was found to have resulted in negligence. This was because the courts went to great lengths to modify the law after accepting that the case would otherwise not successfully provide compensation to the patient on the basis of the orthodox negligence equation.

The common law approach does, however, show autonomy to be a primarily negative concept by respecting the patient's right to *refuse* treatment as in *St George's Healthcare NHS Trust v S; R v Collins and others, ex parte S* [1998] 3 All ER 673 but not the right to *demand* lawful treatment.

Obtaining valid informed consent for proposed treatment from patients, their parent or guardian, as appropriate, is a COPDEND curriculum competency[125] that you are expected to demonstrate during FT. In *Standards for the Dental Team*, the GDC has adopted the term 'valid consent' as opposed to 'informed consent', presumably since the giving of information, or the one-off event of signing a form, does not constitute proper consent. Rather, for consent to be valid you must include making the following considerations:

- Determining whether your patient has the capacity to consent. The Mental Capacity Act 2005 creates a statutory test for capacity which asks the question whether the person in question is unable to make a specific decision when they need to. The Act provides that a person is unable to make a decision for him/herself if he/she is unable to: understand the information relevant to the decision; retain that information; use the information as part of the decision-making process; or communicate his decision by any means, including sign language.
- Gaining parental consent for minors or considering whether they are deemed to be 'Gillick competent' by assessing their capacity to consent.
- Acting in your patient's 'best interests' when you deem them not to have the capacity to consent. Determining what is in your patient's best

---

125 Committee of Postgraduate Dental Deans and Directors UK (COPDEND). *Interim Dental Foundation Training Curriculum & Assessment Framework Guidance 2013–2014*. Oxford: COPDEND; 2013. Clinical domain, ¶2 (5).

interests is not the same as a paternalistic 'dentist knows best' approach. The entitlement of a patient to be treated in their best interests, as supported by Section 4(6) of the Mental Capacity Act 2005, considers the beliefs and values that would be likely to influence a patient's decision if they had capacity.

- Finding out what your patient wants to know, in what format, as well as what you think they need to know. Things that your patient might want to know include: options for treatment, the risks and the potential benefits; why you think a particular treatment is necessary and appropriate for them; the consequences, risks and benefits of the treatment you propose; the likely prognosis; your recommended option; the cost of the proposed treatment; the proposed costs of future treatment should complications arise; what might happen if the proposed treatment is not carried out; and whether the treatment is guaranteed, how long it is guaranteed for and any exclusions that may apply.

- Checking that your patient has understood the information you have given, been able to express any concerns and have had their queries fully answered.

- Providing your patient with reasonable time to consider the treatment options in order to make a decision. Also encouraging your patients who have communication difficulties to have somebody with them to help them ask questions or understand your answers.

- Documenting the discussions you have had with your patient in the process of gaining consent since it is these discussions that determine whether the consent is valid. It is often a good idea to involve your dental nurse in the record-keeping process to remind you of any important discussions that took place with the patient. Information, such as risks, *specific* to your patient should be documented in the records which is a better approach than relying on the use of generic consent forms. Please remember that the NHS FP17DC form is not a satisfactory way of demonstrating valid consent.

 READING POINT! You can access the *FGDP Clinical Examination and Record-Keeping: good practice guidelines.* 2nd edition at: www.fgdp.org.uk/content/publications/clinical-examination-and-record-keeping-good-pract.ashx

Running into difficulties

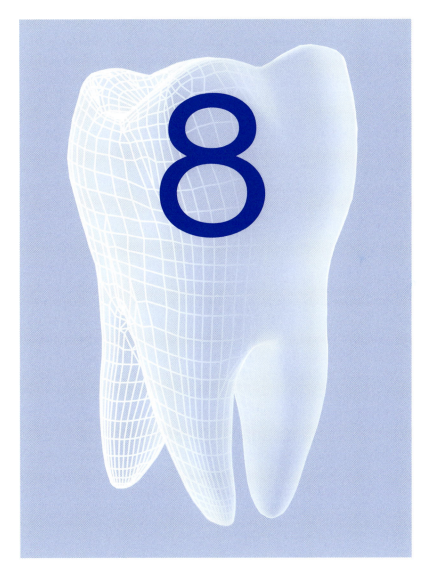

8

ETHICS

Being law-abiding is a behaviour expected of you as a professional and the law is fairly black and white in telling you what to do and what not to do. However, in some cases the law leaves a grey area and it is on these occasions that doing the right thing will only come naturally if you make ethical decisions. This is demonstrated by the fact that the GDC's powers extend to enforcing sanctions against your registration even when no law has been broken. 'Ethics' relate to the moral code guiding our behaviour, whether this is from the GDC or the Seven Principles of Public Life enunciated by the Nolan Committee. An awareness of the ethical or moral aspect to one's conduct together with the urge to prefer right over wrong is considered as being your conscience, something which you should be guided by. Ethical behaviour is not old fashioned or fuddy-duddy but rather rewarding and respectful of the society that we live within, let alone mandatory for remaining on the GDC's register. Understanding and applying the principles of ethical behaviour relevant to dentistry, including honesty, confidentiality, personal and professional integrity and appropriate moral values, is a COPDEND curriculum competency[126] that you are expected to demonstrate during FT.

Conscience is the inner voice that warns us somebody may be looking.

—HL Mencken (1880–1956)

MOTIVATION

It is not uncommon to experience a lack of motivation during the year. This could be considered as the lack of a desire either to learn or to work. If you lack the desire to learn or engage with learning it is likely that there is one or a combination of inhibiting factors blocking your learning (*see* Table 8.1).

---

126 Committee of Postgraduate Dental Deans and Directors UK (COPDEND). *Interim Dental Foundation Training Curriculum & Assessment Framework Guidance 2013–2014.* Oxford: COPDEND; 2013. Professionalism domain, ¶1 (2).

TABLE 8.1 Learning-inhibiting factors and their solutions

Factor	Type	Solution
Assessments used to assess your progress	Extrinsic	Better understand the precise ways that you will be assessed throughout the year by asking your ES and FTPD
Relevance of teaching	Extrinsic	If you perceive the teaching not to be relevant to your stage of learning, you should feed this back to your ES or FTPD
Previous experience	Intrinsic	If past experience is associated with certain emotions blocking your learning, it is important that you try to discuss this with your ES
Learning style does not match with teaching style	Intrinsic	Work with your ES to discover your preferred learning style using Honey and Mumford's Learning Styles Questionnaire
Relationship with ES or FTPD	Extrinsic	Tactfully try to raise any issues directly with your ES or FTPD, or, failing this, with the Associate Director of Foundation Training
Educational environment, such as the location of in-practice tutorials	Extrinsic	Bring this to the attention of your ES, explaining you feel that the environment is not conducive to your learning

SEEKING HELP

A 2012 survey conducted by Cardiff University revealed that over a fifth of trainers reported concerns with their FD knowing when to seek help and advice.[127] Knowing when to seek help and advice from your ES is a skill fundamental to patient safety and your professional development. Common reasons for not seeking help and their potential remedies are listed in Table 8.2.

---

127 Gilmour A, Jones R, Bullock AD. *Dental Foundation Trainers' Expectations of a Dental Graduate*. Final Report. Cardiff: Wales Deanery/Cardiff University; 2012. p. 58.

TABLE 8.2 Reasons for not seeking help and their remedies

Cause	Solution
Not being fully aware of your limitations	Reflecting upon suboptimal clinical outcomes to identify the gaps in your knowledge and/or skills
Not being fully aware when a procedure is heading towards an unsuccessful outcome	Identifying the warning signs and learning to become more aware of them
Uncomfortable asking ES for help	Reflecting upon why you feel uncomfortable. Is it because of the feedback previously received or perhaps because there is seldom the opportunity to speak in confidence?
Inability to ask ES for help	This could perhaps be due to barriers preventing you from accessing your ES. Try raising this concern directly with your ES

HEALTH ISSUES

Should you have or develop health concerns during FT you should not keep these to yourself, as they may act to hamper your progress and ultimately risk patient safety. You should raise any health concerns, or suspected health concerns, with your FTPD in the first instance – your FTPD can provide guidance on managing your health concern in the context of your attendance and assessment. Your employer may signpost you to the practice's local NHS occupational health service, and you may wish to access further information through the NHS Health for Work Adviceline website at: www.health4work. nhs.uk.

POSTURE PERFECT

A contributing factor to chronic back and neck pain is poor posture, and a staggering 60%–80% of dentists experience chronic back and neck pain.[128] It is common for dentists to put themselves last regarding comfort while treating patients – as you twist your body around on your dental stool when trying to get an optimal view of the oral cavity, and then holding yourself in that same position for the duration of the appointment. A more effective approach would be to firstly get yourself into an optimal and comfortable position for your body and subsequently position your patient to best suit you. Your patient plans to sit in the dental chair for just a matter of minutes,

---

128 Mangharam J, McGlothan JD. Ergonomics and Dentistry: a literature review. In: Murphy DC, editor. *Ergonomics and the Dental Care Worker.* Washington, DC: American Public Health Association; 1998.

while you plan to rely on your neck and back being asymptomatic through your practising career. It is important that you look after your back by regularly visiting a chiropractor.

 TIP! You could invest in a stool that supports your posture while you work, such as a saddle stool, which encourages you to sit in a saddle posture by lowering the thighs, opening the hips and positioning the spine into a healthy lordotic curve.

SHARPEN THE SAW

Habit 7 in Stephen Covey's *The 7 Habits of Highly Effective People: Powerful Lessons in Personal Change*[129] is 'Sharpen the Saw'. Covey uses the analogy of a woodcutter who is sawing continuously but who meanwhile is becoming less productive, because the process of cutting dulls the blade. The solution for the woodcutter is to periodically sharpen the saw. Comparatively, if your productivity begins to decrease, you should 'sharpen the saw of your life'. This is not just achieved through doing nothing, as this may involve resting the saw altogether, but through having a balance within the following areas:
- *dentistry* – for your skills and knowledge
- *exercise* – for your physical body
- *spiritualisation* – for your mind and motivation
- *socialisation* – for your emotions and capacity for enjoyment.

PROGRESS

Your clinical, academic and emotional progress throughout the year is carefully and continuously monitored through in-practice assessments and through all contact with your ES, FTPD, Associate Director of Foundation Training and Director of Postgraduate Dental Education and Training. Despite this, you may still feel that you are not ready to practise unsupervised at the end of the year, or you may not feel as competent or proficient in certain clinical skills as you would like. If this is the case, you have a responsibility to inform your ES and FTPD as well as documenting these concerns in e-PDP so that these weaknesses can be improved upon, possibly with remedial training.

---

129 Covey SR. *The 7 Habits of Highly Effective People: powerful lessons in personal change.* New York: Simon & Schuster; 1989.

THE FD–ES RELATIONSHIP

Your relationship with your ES should be open, honest and one of mutual respect. If you should encounter any difficulties with the training practice facilities or staff, then you should be able to discuss these with your ES, or practice owner, in the hope that they can be remedied. Issues with your ES, however, can be more difficult to broach, but you must try to resolve any concerns you have by discussing them directly with your trainer in the first instance. If you do not feel comfortable doing so, or if the situation does not improve, then you should inform your FTPD or Associate Director of Foundation Training. All allegations are thoroughly and objectively explored by speaking separately with you and your ES. You must bear in mind that a practice is unlikely to be allocated another FD, or conversely it is unlikely that you shall be allocated an alternative training practice merely because the current arrangements are not to your/your ES's liking.

It can be possible for your training experience to be affected by your ES not meeting the responsibilities expected of him or her. Examples of this can include if your ES:

- works for fewer than 3 days per week in the same premises as you, in a surgery to which you have good access
- does not provide you with adequate administrative support and the full-time assistance of a suitably experienced dental nurse
- does not provide satisfactory facilities (including an adequate supply of handpieces and instruments, sufficient to allow them to be sterilised between patients) and relevant opportunities so that a wide range of NHS practice is experienced and so far as is reasonably possible so that you are fully occupied
- is not available for guidance in both clinical and administrative matters: does not provide help on request or where necessary
- does not prepare and conduct hourly tutorials on a weekly basis (within normal practice hours).

It is easy to assume that by raising a concern you could strain your relationship with your ES or alternatively you could risk extending your year should you need to be reallocated to another training practice, but this is incorrect. If you fail to raise any concerns that you may have, these will not improve and you could hamper your progress as well as possibly risk patient safety.

ERRORS

A medical error can be considered to be a preventable adverse effect of care, whether or not it is evident or harmful to the patient. Medical errors have been described as human errors in healthcare.[130] You should not practise defensively for error avoidance, otherwise you will never be able to identify areas for improvement. We learn from failure, not from success, so you should never be afraid to make errors.

Anyone who has never made a mistake has never tried anything new.

—Albert Einstein (1879–1955)

The Swiss cheese model,[131] proposed by James Reason, has become one of the dominant paradigms for analysing medical errors. Any error or weakness has the potential likelihood to compromise patient safety, but, according to this metaphor, hazards are prevented from causing adverse outcomes by a series of barriers. Each barrier has unintended weaknesses, or holes – hence the metaphor of Swiss cheese. When all holes are simultaneously aligned, the hazard reaches the patient and causes harm.

While the particular sequence of events may never be repeated, the various contributing factors can come together on particular occasions in configurations that can result in error. The strength of deconstructing incidents into these component elements lies in the fact that, once identified, preventive strategies can be applied.

So if we consider performing an extraction, for instance, it is more likely that the patient's incorrect tooth is extracted if all of the following barriers are simultaneously breached:

- *Barrier 1 (Examination and History)*: inadequate information collected regarding which tooth is problematic, and no diagnosis is recorded
- *Barrier 2 (Communication)*: treatment options or a plan are not discussed with the patient; therefore, there is no confirmation of the treatment to be conducted
- *Barrier 3 (Key Policies and Procedures)*: no radiographic justification or evaluation is recorded
- *Barrier 4: (Teamwork)*: the dental nurse provides the incorrect extraction forceps for the procedure.

130 Zhang J, Patel VL, Johnson TR. Medical error: is the solution medical or cognitive? *J Am Med Inform Assoc.* 2008; 6(Suppl. 1): S75–7.
131 Reason J. Human error: models and management. *BMJ.* 2000; **320**: 768–70.

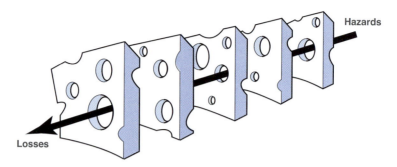

FIGURE 8.1 Illustration of the Swiss cheese model

STRESS

Workplace stress can leave us more vulnerable to receiving complaints through affecting patient interaction and an increased likelihood of us making mistakes. It has been proven that GDPs suffer from work-related stress, with the fragility of the dentist–patient relationship being one of the main factors, alongside time and scheduling pressures.[132]

Running late is a risk factor for adverse incidents, because of the impact on the clinician and partly because of the impact upon the patient's perception of the care that he or she is about to receive. Therefore, often when running late the safest thing to do is to stop and decide which patients could potentially be deferred for another time if possible. However, this must be left as the last resort, as clearly it will be inconvenient for patients, especially if it is at short notice.

Evidence suggests an uncomfortable truth about our profession: the suicide rate is higher among dentists than those in other occupations.[133] It is difficult to identify specific triggers of stress, as we all have different trigger points, but the stress associated with threats against our career can be difficult to manage without support. Although sometimes it may feel like the whole of the profession has turned against you, you must remember that there are individuals and organisations who exist to support you in a non-judgemental way. In fact, mentoring is about the support gained from others who have a personal experience of the problems that you are encountering.

---

132 Myers HL, Myers LB. 'It's difficult being a dentist': stress and health in the general dental practitioner. *Br Dent J.* 2004; **197**(2): 89–93. Discussion 83; quiz 100–1.

133 Sancho FM, Ruiz CN. Risk of suicide amongst dentists: myth or reality? *Int Dent J.* 2010; **60**(6): 411–18.

TIP! You can access support from the following sources:
- LETB mentoring and counselling
- a Practitioner Advice and Support Scheme group
- your LDC
- the BDA.

THE CONSEQUENCES MODEL

Negative consequences associated with dental treatment can range from a patient losing a tooth to a patient suffering a life-threatening medical emergency. The consequences model[134] is traditionally used to encourage bold decision-making, but here we will consider how the extent of the negative consequences of your decisions relates to the extent of your knowledge and skills.

In the first few months of FT you may find yourself deciding whether to perform specific procedures that you may not have performed in months because of clinical inactivity after graduating, thereby rendering your knowledge base and skills dormant. The risks associated with performing such procedures based upon having inadequate knowledge and skills are high, having far-reaching consequences for patients in terms of their safety. If in doubt, it is always safer to obtain a second opinion from your ES, or, in the worst-case scenario, to either refer or defer a decision. Not making a decision is a decision in itself. As Figure 8.2 shows, when your knowledge and certainty in performing procedures increases, your decisions become better informed and negative consequences diminish.

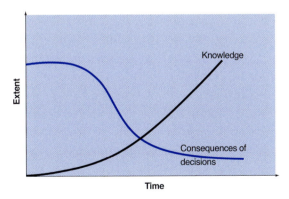

FIGURE 8.2 The consequences model

---

134 Nimmons S. *Enterprise Architecture Patterns: the bold decision maker*. 2011. Available at: http://stevenimmons.org/2011/12/enterprise-architecture-patterns-the-bold-decision-maker/ (accessed November 2013).

Survival guide

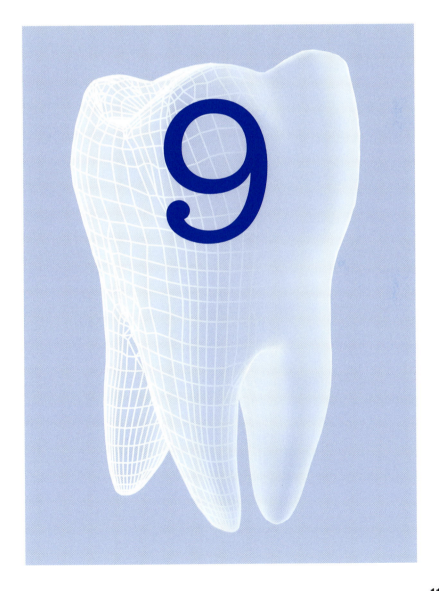

NEW SKILLS AND TECHNIQUES

There remains some variance between clinical procedures taught at under-graduate level and those used in general dental practice. An example is the use of amalgam restorations to restore posterior teeth. Although amalgam remains the main restorative material in NHS practice in the UK, its teaching has reduced in many UK dental schools.[135] This means that during FT you may be taught and expected to perform new clinical skills, meaning that you will be expected to go back to being a *novice* before going on to develop *safe beginner* status.

AWARENESS AND RESPONSIBILITY

Awareness and responsibility have been found to be the common factors among the world's top performing athletes, as researched by David Hemery for his book *Sporting Excellence: What Makes a Champion?*.[136] These are also important factors for a successful FD.

- *Awareness* of your training needs (*conscious incompetence*) through self-reflection is important in helping you to improve your knowledge and skills throughout FT. Awareness will also help you to prevent suboptimal outcomes from recurring since reflective practice builds competence. Awareness also captures how well 'in touch' you are with the outcome, which for all of us is the patient at the end of the process. For instance, while operating a handpiece you receive various inputs, such as the whirring sound, the tactile nature of the rotating bur and patient feedback about the water generated. No matter how fast you might be at reacting to changes in any of these inputs, you will be unable to create the desired outcome of a successful crown preparation and a satisfied patient unless you are able to identity and act upon each individual input.
- *Responsibility* is influenced by choice. In the FT year you are encouraged to immerse yourself into learning and experiencing as many clinical procedures as possible, using this unique platform as a springboard to launch you into your career. But the alternative option is to do enough to simply meet your obligations, merely using the FT experience as a stepping stone in your career. The choice is yours.

---

135 Lynch CD, Frazier KB, McConnell RJ, *et al*. State-of-the-art techniques in operative dentistry: contemporary teaching of posterior composites in UK and Irish dental schools. *Br Dent J*. 2010; **209**(3): 129–36.
136 Hemery D. *Sporting Excellence: what makes a champion?* London: Collins Willow; 1991.

CONSUMER SERVICE

As an FD you are supplied patients to see by your training practice, but this supply is not endless and very much depends upon how satisfied patients are with the treatment and service that you provide. Without patients our roles would be defunct, therefore the service element in dentistry is important and you should try to extend the service you provide that little bit further each time you see a patient. Service is also important from a reputational perspective in that patients will tell more people if they are dissatisfied than if they are not. This was demonstrated in research conducted by Coca-Cola in 1981[137] where it was found that a median of as many as 9–10 people will hear about a consumer's negative experience whereas a median of only 4–5 people will hear about a positive experience.

The 'patient empowerment' movement is gathering pace in NHS dentistry. This movement encourages patients to be more informed about their care, have greater access and have greater control over their care, which are themes proven to be successful in the consumer setting. Patients are considered as consumers as opposed to customers because they are the users of a product or service. In the consumerisation of dentistry it is important not to lose sight of the fact that patients are often not seeking to use dentistry because they *want* to but rather because they *need* to in order to resolve a problem. Also important is the fact that unlike consumers the decision-making process for patients is more involved since they are required to absorb technical information during a time of anxiety.

NHS REGULATIONS

It is unlikely that you would have been taught much about the NHS regulations at undergraduate level, but in your FT year you are expected to have a firm grasp of these regulations. Briefly, the NHS regulations refer to:
- the National Health Service (General Dental Services Contracts) Regulations 2005, and
- the National Health Service (Dental Charges) Regulations 2005 and the National Health Service (Dental Charges) Amendment Regulations 2006.

---

137 Customer Information Centre, The Coca-Cola Company. *Measuring the Grapevine: consumer response and word-of-mouth.* Conducted for the Corporate Consumer Affairs Department of The Coca-Cola Company by Technical Assistance Research Programs Inc, The Coca-Cola Company; 1981. p. 4.

Although your ES will provide you with one-to-one teaching around this topic, which will be supplemented by your scheme's study day programme, FDs have felt it beneficial to gain further information about the NHS regulations. You can gain further information from the following resources:

- NHS BSA Dental Services website (www.nhsbsa.nhs.uk/DentalServices. aspx)
- D'Cruz L, Rattan R, Watson M, *Understanding NHS Dentistry: Preparing for the Future* (2nd revised edition, Dental Publishing, 2010)
- Department of Health, *Guide to NHS Dental Services in England*, 2009.

WORKING ELSEWHERE

Clause 17.6 of the Foundation Training contract outlines that unless part of FT the FD should *'not normally attend any patient or perform any operation or prosthetic work for any person other than the Practice'.* If you are considering employment in addition to your Foundation Training contract you must first gain written approval of both your ES and the director of postgraduate dental education. They will consider whether this would impinge on your commitment and ability to complete FT.

You must also bear in mind that, as laid down in the NHS (Performers Lists) (England) Regulations 2013, you give an undertaking not to perform any primary dental services except when acting for and under the direction of your trainer (ES).[138]

GIFTS

As outlined in the GDC's *Standards for the Dental Team*:[139]

> You must refuse any gifts, payment or hospitality if accepting them could affect, or could appear to affect, your professional judgment.

Some dentists feel that accepting gifts from patients will always ultimately prejudice their professional judgement so they maintain a policy of never accepting gifts from patients. The National Health Service (General Dental

---

138 The NHS (Performers Lists) (England) Regulations 2013, ¶33 3(a)(i).
139 General Dental Council. *Standards for the Dental Team*. London: General Dental Council; 2013. Standard 1.7.5.

Services Contracts) Regulations 2005 outlines a requirement for a register of gifts to be kept for gifts of an individual value of more than £100.00.[140]

HOLIDAYS

Clause 19 of the Foundation Contract outlines your entitlement to 5.6 weeks' holiday, including bank holidays, with full pay during the period of 12 months in the practice. The dates of these holidays are to be agreed and booked with your ES, and must not be during a study day. If you agree to work on a public holiday, you will be given a day's leave in lieu. Be careful not to take more holidays than the 5.6 weeks allowable, otherwise a deduction can be made from your final pay on a pro rata basis at the date of termination, as outlined in clause 21 of the Foundation Contract.

Please note, as outlined in clause 19 of the Foundation Contract, you should not take more than 3 days' annual leave within the first 8 weeks of the training year without the written approval of the Postgraduate Dental Dean or Director of Postgraduate Education.

MISSING STUDY DAYS

It is unlikely that you will receive your scheme's study day programme for the entire year in advance as some days can only be planned once the collective learning needs of the scheme are identified. Under these circumstances there is an expectation for you not to book any holidays until you know the study day dates. Even then, there is a risk that unscheduled study day dates may arise, which you would be expected to attend.

Sometimes, however, there may be an unavoidable reason for missing a study day, such as illness. Furthermore, clause 17.8 of the Foundation Contract outlines that there are exceptional circumstances when you can absent yourself from a study day, but that this must be supported by a written application made at least 6 weeks in advance to the FTPD and Director of Postgraduate Education.

If you miss a study day then you will usually be expected to make it up with suitable equivalent training/education attended in your own time and at your own cost.

---

140 The NHS (General Dental Services Contracts) Regulations 2005 P6 S3 P10, ¶83 (1).

SICKNESS

There is no paid sick leave within the contract. Therefore, only statutory sick pay (SSP) is payable if you have been absent from work through illness. In order to be considered for SSP, you must notify your employer of the illness, who is entitled to ask for reasonable evidence of incapacity, such as self-certification, for periods of illness lasting fewer than 7 days, or a doctor's note for illnesses of 7 days or longer. If you are sick for 3 calendar days in a row or fewer, this is not covered by SSP.

If you miss a study day because of illness then you will usually be expected to make it up with suitable equivalent training/education attended in your own time and at your own cost.

WORKING HOURS

Clause 18 of the Foundation Contract outlines an expectation for you to work 35 hours a week exclusive of lunch breaks, and this includes any scheme study days. This is most predictably distributed as 9 a.m.–5 p.m. Monday–Friday, with 1 hour for lunch. The opening hours of your practice, however, may require you to work differently – for instance, late evenings, Saturdays or not working on the days when you have no study day planned. The best way for you and your ES to ensure that you are working the right amount of cumulative hours over the year is by using the following calculation:

46.4 weeks × 35 hours/week = 1624 total hours for the year
(inclusive of study days)

PERFORMING PRIVATE DENTISTRY

There is an expectation for FDs to predominantly perform NHS dentistry within the NHS, although there are situations where the need to provide Private treatment may arise, such as treatment for cosmetic purposes. Where an FD provides private treatment, the fees would be accrued to the practice and not the FD, as stipulated in clause 17.3 of the Foundation Contract.

TOOTH WHITENING

Tooth whitening is available on the NHS as long as there is appropriate clinical justification, such as the discolouration of an anterior tooth as a result of disease process which may otherwise compromise the social confidence of a patient. If demanded as a result of an ageing or staining process, tooth whitening would rather be deemed as a cosmetic, and therefore private, treatment. Under the Cosmetic Products (Safety) (Amendment) Regulations 2012 dental professionals can legally treat patients over 18 years of age with tooth whitening treatments which contain or release up to 6% hydrogen peroxide (or 16% carbamide peroxide). These regulations apply to the whitening of vital or non-vital teeth and regardless of whether the discolouration resulted from a disease, ageing or staining process. The first cycle of treatment should be administered by a dentist or be carried out under their supervision, after which the treatment can then be completed by the patient at home. Prior to embarking on a course of tooth whitening you must carry out an examination to determine whether tooth whitening is suitable for the patient, documenting this along with the consent process (*see* Chapter 7).

FACIAL AESTHETICS

The UK facial aesthetics market has grown in recent years, and includes treatments such as the use of injectable botulinum toxin (Botox is a brand name) and non-permanent dermal fillers, for cosmetic or non-cosmetic purposes. Indeed, some of the medically related uses of botulinum toxin include temporomandibular joint pain disorders and excessive salivation. Although facial aesthetic procedures are provided by a variety of professionals, dentists are well placed to carry out these procedures safely because of their knowledge and standards. The GDC have recognised that providing non-surgical cosmetic injectables is within the scope of practice of a dentist as an additional skill that he or she could develop,[141] usually after further and appropriate training with adequate indemnity cover.

In a year in which you are learning and practising orthodox dental skills, however, performing facial aesthetic procedures would not be appropriate for two reasons. First, because these procedures pose a certain level of risk to you based on your unfamiliarity resulting from limited training and supervision, not to mention your relative unfamiliarity in dealing with the high expectations demanded of the typical patient demographic. Second, performing facial aesthetic procedures would not be appropriate during an NHS funded training scheme.

---

141 General Dental Council. *Scope of Practice*. London: General Dental Council; 2013. p. 11.

IMPLANT DENTISTRY

The provision of implants is an additional skill[142] that dentists can develop during their career with further and appropriate training. Most dentists are attracted to the financial returns associated with placing implants, but also associated with this are the increased risks of complaints arising from sub-optimal outcomes. There are generally three main ways to get involved with dental implants:

1. treatment planning and referring appropriate cases
2. restoring implants after being surgically placed by an appropriately qualified colleague
3. treatment planning, placing and restoring dental implants.

Understanding the principles and techniques involved in the surgical placement of dental implants is a COPDEND curriculum competency[143] that you are expected to demonstrate during FT. However, considering the time it takes to acquire the competence and confidence in placing dental implants it is likely that you will only be able to understand how to treatment plan for cases during FT. If you develop an interest in dental implants after FT, however, it is recommended that you explore this through further qualifications, such as a postgraduate diploma or Master's programme, and working under the supervision of an experienced mentor.

JURY SERVICE

If you are sent a jury summons, you should apply to the court for deferral on the grounds that you are on a training course for a period of 12 months. Jury service usually lasts for up to 10 working days – but can be longer, thereby risking your progress in FT. If the court does not grant deferral, please inform your FTPD, who will support your appeal against this decision.

I-DENTISTRY

We live in the information age, characterised by our ability to transfer information freely and to have instant access to information by virtue of the internet. Many devices now enable us to access the internet, including smart phones,

---

142 General Dental Council. *Scope of Practice*. London: General Dental Council; 2013. p. 11.
143 Committee of Postgraduate Dental Deans and Directors UK (COPDEND). *Interim Dental Foundation Training Curriculum & Assessment Framework Guidance 2013–2014*. Oxford: COPDEND; 2013. Clinical domain, ¶7 (4).

so that we can communicate across the world with the click of a button. Social media, including social networking, is an excellent way to keep in touch with friends and family but caution must be taken with what you publish in this very public arena. Consider your social media profile and the content of the information you choose to share publically, because photographs can easily be manipulated and your comments taken out of context. To quote the film *The Social Network*,[144] 'the internet isn't written in pencil … it's written in ink' – indelible ink.

You should take note of standard 9.1.3 in the GDC's *Standards for the Dental Team*:

> You should not publish anything that could affect patients' and the public's confidence in you, or the dental profession, in any public media, unless this is done as part of raising a concern. In particular, you must not make personal, inaccurate or derogatory comments about patients or colleagues.

You must also be careful not to disclose patient-identifiable information, even if using professional social media for the purpose of discussing best practice.

LOUPES

Loupes are a key tool required to conduct a comprehensive examination. Their main benefit is that they enlarge the working image, thereby allowing you to observe structures not easily visible to the naked eye. Practically, magnification also allows better procedural precision – for example, during crown preparation or caries removal. The level of magnification depends upon the type of procedure being undertaken. For general dental procedures, ×2.5 to ×3.5 magnifications are usually sufficient; while for crown and bridgework and for endodontics, higher magnifications of ×4.5 and ×6.0 may be desired. The most effective way to measure the effectiveness of a magnification system is to try it on your own practice. Many companies will offer free trial periods to try out loupes; whenever possible, take advantage of these trial periods to determine the best system for you. The cost of purchasing dental loupes can be justified by improvements to diagnosis and operative treatment.[145] Loupes can also help in keeping an ideal working posture by being configured to ensure the maintenance of an appropriate working distance to maintain focus.

---

144 *The Social Network*. Film. Directed by Fincher D, USA. Columbia Pictures; 2010.
145 James T, Gilmour AS. Magnifying loupes in modern dental practice: an update. *Dent Update*. 2010; **37**(9): 633–6.

When purchasing loupes you should select ones in which the convergence angles are precisely aligned and permanently fixed. Loupes take time to acclimatise to and within the first fortnight of wearing them it is generally recommended to restrict their use to an hour for each session.

PROJECT WORK: PORTFOLIO OF EVIDENCE

The completion of FT usually includes FDs being required to produce a portfolio[146] containing a collection of evidence where you would reflect on your professional development in five core clinical and management skill areas. The FT portfolio of evidence provides a way of you demonstrating several curriculum competencies[147] during FT and acts to assist you in preparing for general professional dental examinations. The FT portfolio of evidence has also been historically helpful for FDs sitting the MJDF examination because the portfolio was assessed for credit towards the examination until 2011.

The requirements for the FT portfolio of evidence are either the same as those for the pre-2011 MJDF requirements[148] or the same as the FGDP (UK) Key Skills in Primary Dental Care[149] (which provides a quality standard endorsed by the FGDP). Due to regional variation you should check the precise requirements for your FT portfolio of evidence with your FTPD.

Pre-2011 MJDF requirements

Of the five key skill areas to be demonstrated, three are core and therefore mandatory and the remaining two are optional out of a choice of five.

Core skills:
- Infection Control
- Radiography and Radiation Protection
- Medical Emergencies.

---

146 COPDEND. Dental Foundation Training Policy Statement, ¶35. Available at: www.copdend.org/content.aspx?Group=foundation&Page=foundation_policystatement (accessed November 2013), ¶39.

147 Committee of Postgraduate Dental Deans and Directors UK (COPDEND). *Interim Dental Foundation Training Curriculum & Assessment Framework Guidance 2013–2014*. Oxford: COPDEND; 2013. Management and leadership domain, ¶2 (8) and ¶2 (9).

148 Diploma of Membership of the Joint Dental Faculties of the Royal College of Surgeons of England. MJDF Portfolio Guide 2010, version 2. MJDF. Available at: www.mjdf.org.uk/docs/portfolio_guide.pdf (accessed November 2013).

149 FGDP (UK). *Key Skills in Primary Dental Care* (CD-ROM). version 2. Smile-on Ltd; 2007.

Optional skills:
- Health and Safety in Clinical Practice
- Record keeping
- Team Work
- Law and Ethics
- Prevention and Dental Public Health.

Key skills in primary dental care requirements

Of the five key skill areas to be demonstrated, three are core and therefore mandatory and the remaining two are optional out of a choice of four.

Core skills:
- Infection Control
- Radiography
- Medical Emergencies.

Optional skills:
- Clinical record keeping
- Legislation and good practice guidelines
- Risk management and communication
- Team training.

Given that the FT portfolio of evidence no longer helps FDs working towards the MJDF qualification, some thought has been given towards possibly changing the format of the FT portfolio to incorporate the CQC essential standards.

PROJECT WORK: CLINICAL AUDIT

Clinical audit has been defined[150] as:

> a quality improvement process that seeks to improve patient care and outcomes through systematic review of care against explicit criteria and the implementation of change. Aspects of the structure, processes, and outcomes of care are selected and systematically evaluated against explicit criteria. Where indicated, changes are implemented at an individual, team, or service level and further monitoring is used to confirm improvement in healthcare delivery.

---

150 National Institute for Clinical Excellence. *Principles for Best Practice in Clinical Audit.* Oxford: Radcliffe Medical Press; 2002.

The conventional way of presenting the clinical audit process is as a 'cycle' and in order for the audit cycle to be closed, changes in practice should be implemented and then re-audited to ascertain whether improvements in service delivery have occurred as a result.[151]

Regularly reviewing the outcomes of treatment given in an effort to provide the highest standards of patient care, and understanding the importance of clinical audit and its regular implementation is a COPDEND curriculum competency[152] that you are expected to demonstrate in FT. The following serves as a practical '10 step guide' for carrying out a clinical audit:

Step 1 – Select your topic
Step 2 – Review the literature
Step 3 – Set the standards
Step 4 – Design the audit
Step 5 – Collect the data
Step 6 – Analyse the data
Step 7 – Feed back findings
Step 8 – Change clinical practice
Step 9 – Review standards
Step 10 – Re-audit

TIP! Try selecting an audit topic which is relevant to your clinical practice rather than focusing on legislative and regulatory required topics such as:
- the quality of radiographs (in conformance with the Ionising Radiation (Medical Exposure) Regulations 2000), and
- the local self-assessment audit for assessing implementation of HTM 01-05: decontamination in primary care dental practices and related infection prevention and control issues.

CASE PRESENTATIONS

Although the format of case presentations varies from scheme to scheme, they generally involve the presentation of a clinical case that you have managed during the course of the FT year. Giving an effective presentation that uses

151 Royal College of Psychiatrists. *Undertaking a Clinical Audit Project: a step-by-step guide*. Available at: www.rcpsych.ac.uk/pdf/clinauditchap2.pdf (accessed November 2013).
152 Committee of Postgraduate Dental Deans and Directors UK (COPDEND). *Interim Dental Foundation Training Curriculum & Assessment Framework Guidance 2013–2014*. Oxford: COPDEND; 2013 professionalism, ¶2 (7).

relevant teaching materials and is targeted to the level of understanding and expectations of the audience is a COPDEND curriculum competency[153] that you are expected to demonstrate during FT.

The following are some tips regarding case presentations.

- Start thinking about selecting possible cases early in the year. Treatment plans could go on for months, so it is better to start sooner rather than later.
- Have several back-up cases available as a contingency in case your primary case patient does not complete his or her treatment for whatever reason.
- Ensure that a camera is always accessible in your surgery, as you never know when an interesting case could walk through your door.
- Anonymise all patient-identifiable details (including information on radiographs and study models) when presenting.
- Clinical photographs help to bring your presentation to life; the higher quality they are the better. Photographs capturing pre and post treatment can be helpful.
- Try not selecting complex cases involving advanced clinical techniques. Remember that you will be assessed against the benchmark of a month 12 FD, not a specialist.
- Why not bring in any study models to aid your presentation? Better still, these could be articulated.
- You may be assessed on your communication and presenting skills but try not to get carried away with using professional software effects – remember that this is a clinical presentation.
- Rehearse the presentation of your case to ensure that you do not go under or over any time limits.
- Set out your treatment plan clearly in a stepwise manner.
- Reflect on the outcome of the case, what you feel went well and what you feel you could have done better.
- Remember when explaining your case that although your ES and you would be very familiar with the case, your audience may not be.
- Be sure not to take any questions as criticisms. If your approach to the case is at variance with somebody, remember that there is usually not one single definitive treatment plan.
- As FT is an NHS funded scheme, expect questions testing your knowledge of NHS rules and regulations.

---

153 Ibid. Management and leadership domain, ¶4 (8).

ARS EST CELARE ARTEM

Dentistry is often described as where 'art meets science', and the Latin phrase *Ars est celare artem* loosely translates as 'Art hides itself'. Essentially the idea is that the truest art lacks overt ingenuity, and that you need to be at a certain level of competence to see it, let alone appreciate it. In some respects this is what the FT year is about – mastering procedures and techniques that produce outcomes which look relatively simple to the untrained eye.

The postoperative radiograph of a well-shaped and well-obturated root canal treatment performed using hand files, for instance, shows an apparent effortlessness revealing a depth of skill and knowledge so inherent that the hand files are nothing more than a basic tool. Try to remember this Latin phrase when tempted to use advanced clinical techniques and equipment (such as rotary endodontic equipment) during the year.

CLAIMS FOR TRAVEL AND SUBSISTENCE

From 1 April 2013, the delegated responsibility for travel and subsistence payments to dentists undertaking verifiable CPD was given to NHS England Area Teams. You can make claims on FP84 forms, which serve as a certificate of attendance and a claim form for both reimbursement of dental travel and subsistence. The form must then be sent to the relevant Area Team, or shared services (if applicable). The FP84 form sets out the rates at which expenses are reimbursed to NHS staff who have to travel in connection with their official duties.[154]

The rates for reimbursement at the time of writing are detailed here.

Overnight allowance
- Actual receipted cost of bed and breakfast up to a maximum of £55.00
- Non-commercial accommodation (e.g. friends or relatives). £25.00

Meal allowance
- Lunch (applicable when more than 5 hours away from the practice including the times between 12 noon and 2 p.m.). £5.00
- Evening Meal (applicable when away from the practice for more than 10 hours after 7 p.m.). £15.00

---

154 Geddes D. Travel and subsistence for dentists undertaking verifiable continuing professional development. *Primary Care Commissioning Newsletter.* 2013; 29 May (5): 1–2. Available at: www.england. nhs.uk/wp-content/uploads/2013/09/pc-newslt-5.pdf (accessed November 2013).

Mileage allowance

- Dentists using their own vehicle (shortest practicable route between place of work and place visited).   £0.24
- Dentists carrying one of more named eligible dentists to the same course.   £0.05

Travel and subsistence reimbursements are usually paid onto the practice owner's contract and will appear against your name on the monthly schedule received from the NHS BSA. It will be necessary for the practice owner to pay you this reimbursement.

SALARY

The FD salary is fixed and calculated from the Statement of Financial Entitlements[155] produced by the Department of Health. As the salary is standardised there is no regional weighting allowance.

Your employer (either your ES or the practice owner) receives gross funding in 12 equal monthly instalments which includes: their trainer's grant, a reimbursement of your salary and service costs covering the costs of employing you. It is through this arrangement that you are usually paid on a monthly basis, with the precise timing each month dependent upon when your employer usually pays his or her staff. If you are struggling for payment in your first month and have not yet been paid by your employer, it is not unreasonable for you to perhaps ask them for an advance.

As an employee you must have tax and NI deducted, as well as superannuation contributions if you chose to opt into the NHS Pension Scheme. Your itemised payslip received every month should show your payment and all deductions every month. Any queries that you have about your pay and deductions should be taken up with your employer. Failing that, you could approach your FTPD or consult with an accountant who may come to speak to your scheme at a study day.

SUPERANNUATION

Superannuation is a form of pension contribution. The government runs the NHS Superannuation scheme. You will eventually receive a pension based broadly on the total contributions paid throughout your working life as a

---

155 Department of Health. General Dental Services Statement of Financial Entitlements P2, ¶8.2 and Personal Dental Services Statement of Financial Entitlements P2, ¶7.2.

dentist in the NHS. You can opt out of the scheme if you wish. However, it is strongly suggested that you seek professional advice before doing so as the NHS Superannuation Scheme generally provides very high levels of cover at relatively low rates.

Superannuation is charged on your gross salary each month and will be deducted by your employer before he or she pays you. The rate of superannuation for FDs, at time of writing, is 9% of the gross salary. You receive tax relief on superannuation paid. This means that as a result you pay less tax on your salary, as superannuation is deducted from the gross salary and tax worked out on the net after superannuation. You also pay fewer NI contributions when you pay superannuation, as you are treated as 'contracted out' of the State Earnings-Related Pension Scheme. Although it is possible to pay additional voluntary contributions into the superannuation scheme, you should seek professional advice before doing so.

PAYE

PAYE is the system that HMRC uses to collect income tax and NI contributions from employees. The tax and NI contributions are deducted throughout the tax year based on your earnings and then paid to HMRC.

If you have been employed in the current tax year you should have been given a P45 by your previous employer, when you left, that shows the tax you have paid and your tax code. This P45 should be provided to your employer. If you have not been employed in the current tax year, your employer will ask you to fill in form P46. If you do not have a tax code, an emergency code will be used. If you start work and are paid, without a tax code, then later receive a correct coding, a tax refund will apply and your next pay cheque will be much higher.

You shall need to supply your NI number to your employer. If, however, you do not have an NI number then you will need to apply for one. Further information is available at www.hmrc.gov.uk/ni/intro/number.htm.

You pay NI contributions to build up your entitlement to certain state benefits. As an employed FD you will pay Class 1 NI contributions at contracted-out rates.

READING POINT!

- You can access further information on tax codes at: www.hmrc.gov. uk/incometax/codes-basics.htm
- You can access further information on NI at: www.hmrc.gov.uk/ni/ intro/basics.htm
- You can access further information on the NHS Pension Scheme at: www.nhsbsa.nhs.uk/pensions

FINANCIAL PLANNING

Most newly qualified dentists will have some sort of debt resulting from their undergraduate studies, ranging from a student loan to money owed to family members. These debts should ideally be prioritised, not according to the size of the loan but to the action that creditors will take to obtain their money. Knowing your monthly FT salary, you should deduct your forecasted monthly expenditure, which will then provide you with an estimation of how much money can be allocated towards paying off your loans. Once debt-free you can then look towards acquiring savings such as in individual savings accounts.

Remember to save money to pay for:

- the GDC registration fee due at point of registration (usually between June and July)
- membership of a dental defence organisation (usually between June and August)
- the GDC annual retention fee, due between November and December
- MJDF or MFDS examination fee (payable in July or January, depending on the date of examination).

INCOME PROTECTION

Income protection is a form of insurance that pays you a regular income should you be unable to work because of illness or injury; it is therefore relied upon to safeguard a reasonable standard of living. Although income protection insurance is not essential, it is recommended. There are various providers of income protection, and you must carefully consider all terms and conditions. In particular 'own occupation' policies are preferable to 'any occupation' policies.

SURVEYS

During the year you will be requested to complete a range of surveys and questionnaires regarding your experience. This includes the annual National Survey of Dental Foundation Trainees conducted by the Advisory Board for Foundation Training in Dentistry, which reports to the Joint Committee for Postgraduate Training in Dentistry. Please comply with these requests in a timely manner, as you have an obligation to give feedback on your experience to improve FT for the next cohort of dentists.

e-PDP DOS AND DON'TS

TABLE 9.1 List of dos and don'ts relating to e-PDP

Do	Don't
Complete the *Participant's details* section as soon as you get your username and password	Upload an inappropriate profile picture
Complete the various sections in the week that they are due to be completed	Play catch-up, as it's easy to fall behind, which could then affect the accuracy of your entries
Send important messages to other FDs, your ES and FTPD via the *My Messages* section, as this will serve as a log of any concerns	Use the *My Messages* section as a social networking system
Reflect on study days by completing the *Reflection on study days* section	Complete the *Reflection on study days* section, or the *Tutorial Log* section, a long time after the event; your entries should be contemporaneous
Complete the *FD's CPD* section, uploading all CPD certificates that you obtain, as e-PDP will allow you to generate a bespoke report detailing your CPD activities	Complete the *Reflection on study days* section unless you attend verifiable CPD courses outside of the study day programme
Make all of your entries, particularly the reflections, relevant, as they serve as a record of your strengths and weaknesses	Write just a few sentences describing an experience (instead, write more content reflecting on the experience)
Add actions to the *FD's PDP* section; to add an item, click *Add PDP item*	Leave actions as *incomplete*, as you must regularly review the *FD's PDP* section

PROJECT WORK

Try not to put off your FT portfolio of evidence and clinical audit requirements until the second half of your training year, as this will be a particularly busy time when you may be preparing for the MJDF or MFDS Part 1 examinations, applying for posts and completing your case presentation. October–December is usually a good time to be getting busy with project work.

INDEMNITY

As a GDC registrant you are required to ensure that there are adequate and appropriate arrangements in place so that patients can claim any compensation they may be entitled to.

For the majority of FDs, the cover you will have in place will be your own dental defence organisation membership, but other types of cover recognised by the GDC are:

- dental defence organisation cover provided by your employer's membership
- professional indemnity insurance held by you or your employer
- NHS/Crown indemnity.

Professional indemnity is not like shopping for car insurance, and you should not make your decision solely on price, as the costs are broadly comparable. Whereas some dental defence organisations offer discretionary indemnity with no extensive exclusion clauses, others offer the security of an insurance policy with the Financial Services Authority, thereby offering legal safeguards for policyholders. Before choosing a provider don't forget to do your research about them, such as reading about their team of advisors, and asking for recommendations from colleagues, as you will want the best help you can get if you run into problems.

UNIFORM

You should check with your training practice whether there is a uniform code that they expect you to adhere to, such as a specific colour or style of uniform. Generally you are expected to wear short-sleeved uniforms, such as scrubs or tunics, that are freshly laundered each day to reduce contamination. You must remember not to wear your uniform outside the practice or to the WC.

 READING POINT! You can access further information on clothing, uniforms and laundry in paragraphs 6.31–6.35 of the Department of Health's *Health Technical Memorandum 01-05: decontamination in primary care dental practices** available at: www.gov.uk/government/publications/decontamination-in-primary-care-dental-practices

* Department of Health. *Health Technical Memorandum 01-05: decontamination in primary care dental practices.* 2nd ed. Leeds: Department of Health; 2013.

GDC FEES

At the point of registration, following graduation, you would have had to pay a registration fee to enter your name onto the dentist register for the first time. This fee retains your name on the register for the remainder of that year until 31 December.

To practise dentistry past 31 December you will need to remain on the dentist register from 1 January the following year, which requires payment of the annual retention fee (ARF). The ARF is not a membership fee; it confirms your registration for the full period it relates to. The deadline for payment is 31 December each year, and it is not possible to pay the ARF in instalments. Approximately 15 working days after your payment has been processed you will receive your Annual Practising Certificate, posted to your registered address.

You can manage your registration and pay for your application to join the register through the online eGDC platform (at www.egdc-uk.org), which also enables you to view your Annual Practising Certificate.

It is important to remember that without an Annual Practising Certificate you cannot practise dentistry, irrespective of whether you are employed to work in an approved training practice.

 BEWARE! Practising dentistry, even for one day, without successfully paying your ARF and receiving subsequent confirmation, is illegal and may necessitate an investigation of your fitness to practise.

EDUCATIONAL RESOURCES

Although the emphasis during FT is on the application rather than the learning of knowledge, you may nevertheless need to fill gaps in your knowledge base through accessing educational resources. Table 9.2 lists some resources that may be useful.

TABLE 9.2 List of educational resources

Material	Resource
Textbooks	BDA Library: www.bda.org/library
	Postgraduate Medical Education Centre library
Journals	*British Dental Journal*: www.nature.com/bdj/index.html
	Dental Update: www.dental-update.co.uk
Current affairs	*Smile-On News*: www.smile-onnews.com
	Dentistry: www.dentistry.co.uk
	The Dentist: www.the-dentist.co.uk
	The Probe: www.dentalrepublic.co.uk/the-probe
Clinical guidelines	NICE: www.nice.org.uk
	Department of Health: www.gov.uk/government/organisations/department-of-health
Interactive e-resources	e-Den: www.e-lfh.org.uk/projects/dentistry
	Smile-On eLearning: www.healthcare-learning.com/elearning
	The Dental Trauma Guide: www.dentaltraumaguide.org
CPD courses	LETB
	BDA branch section
	LDC

 TIP! Download the official NICE *British National Formulary* (BNF) app for free to access the most up-to-date prescribing information from the BNF at the touch of a button.

LAST BUT NOT LEAST

Foundation Training provides you with the unique opportunity to build upon your undergraduate dental experience within a protected environment. It is regarded by so many dentists as a rite of passage which is presumably why it has been referred to as 'the jewel in the crown' of NHS dentistry.[156] So take every opportunity you can to learn, ask questions and to practise. There is something very special about the synergy created during FT study days which comes from sharing experiences and having fun, so don't forget to enjoy yourself.

---

156 Rattan R. Duty of care. *Dentist magazine*. 2011; **27**(4).

Abbreviations

A'DEP'T	Dental Evaluation of Performance Tool
ARF	Annual retention fee
BDA	British Dental Association
BLS	Basic life support
BSA	Business Services Authority
COPDEND	UK Committee of Postgraduate Dental Deans and Directors
COSHH	Control of substances hazardous to health
CPD	Continuing professional development
CQC	Care Quality Commission
CV	Curriculum vitae
D-CbD	Dental Case-based Discussion
DCT	Dental Core Training
DES	Dentist with Enhanced Skills
e-PDP	Electronic Personal Development Plan
ES	Educational Supervisor
ESPR	Early Stage Peer Review
FD	Foundation Dentist
FGDP	Faculty of General Dental Practice
FT	Foundation Training
FTPD	Foundation Training programme director
GDC	General Dental Council
GDP	General dental practitioner
GIC	Glass ionomet cement
HEE	Health Education England
HMRC	HM Revenue and Customs
LDC	Local dental committee
LETB	Local education and training board
LPN	Local professional network
MFD	Membership of the Faculty of Dentistry
MFDS	Membership of the Faculty of Dental Surgery
MJDF	Membership of the Joint Dental Faculties
NHS	National Health Service
NI	National Insurance
NICE	National Institute for Health and Care Excellence
OMFS	Oral and maxillofacial surgery

OSCE	Objective Structured Clinical Examination
PAQ	Patient Assessment Questionnaire
PAT	Peer assessment tool
PAYE	Pay As You Earn
PDP	Personal Development Plan
RSD	Root surface debridement
SSP	Statutory sick pay
StR	Specialty registrar
TAB	Team assessment of behaviours
UDA	Unit of Dental Activity
UK	United Kingdom
WPBA	Workplace-based assessment

References

Ausubel D, Novak J, Hanesian H. *Educational Psychology: a cognitive view.* 2nd ed. New York, NY: Holt, Rinehart, & Winston; 1978.

Beauchamp TL, Childress JF. *Principles of Biomedical Ethics.* 4th ed. Oxford University Press; 1994.

Bligh DA. *What's the Use of Lectures?* San Francisco, CA: Jossey-Bass; 2000.

Boehler ML, Rogers DA, Schwind CJ, *et al.* An investigation of medical student reactions to feedback: a randomised controlled trial. *Med Educ.* 2006; **40**(8): 746–9.

British Dental Trade Association. *Perceptions of Dentistry and Motivation Research.* Chesham: British Dental Trade Association; Online poll of 5589 UK respondents aged between 18 and 55; April 2012.

Bunting RF Jr, Benton J, Morgan WD. Practical risk management principles for physicians. *J Healthc Risk Manag.* 1998; **18**(4): 29–53.

Care Quality Commission. *Guidance about Compliance: essential standards of quality and safety.* London: Care Quality Commission; 2010.

Csíkszentmihályi M. *Beyond Boredom and Anxiety: experiencing flow in work and play.* 25th Anniversary Edition. San Francisco, CA: Jossey-Bass; 2000.

Committee of Postgraduate Dental Deans and Directors UK (COPDEND). *A Curriculum for UK Dental Foundation Programme Training.* Oxford: COPDEND; 2007.

Committee of Postgraduate Dental Deans and Directors UK (COPDEND). *Dental Foundation Training Policy Statement.* Available at: www.copdend.org/content.aspx?Group=foundation&Page=foundation_policystatement

Committee of Postgraduate Dental Deans and Directors UK (COPDEND). *Dental Foundation Training Portfolio & Assessment: user guide.* Available at: www.copdend.org/data/files/Foundation/Dental%20Foundation%20Training%20Portfolio%20User%20Guide%5B1%5D.pdf

Committee of Postgraduate Dental Deans and Directors UK (COPDEND). *Guidance Notes on the Foundation Contract.* Revised. Oxford: COPDEND; 2013.

Committee of Postgraduate Dental Deans and Directors UK (COPDEND). *Interim Dental Foundation Training Curriculum & Assessment Framework Guidance 2013–2014.* Oxford: COPDEND; 2013.

Committee of Postgraduate Dental Deans and Directors UK (COPDEND). *A Reference Guide for Postgraduate Dental Specialty Training in the UK: The Dental Gold Guide.* 3rd ed. Oxford: COPDEND; 2013.

Covey SR. *The 7 Habits of Highly Effective People: powerful lessons in personal change.* New York: Simon & Schuster; 1989.

Customer Information Centre, The Coca-Cola Company. *Measuring the Grapevine: consumer response and word-of-mouth,* conducted for the Corporate Consumer Affairs

Department of The Coca-Cola Company by Technical Assistance Research Programs Inc, The Coca-Cola Company; 1981. p. 4.

Darzi A. Quality and the NHS Next Stage Review. *Lancet.* 2008; **371**(9624): 1563–4.

Department of Health. *A First Class Service: quality in the new NHS.* London: Department of Health; 1998.

Department of Health. *Delivering Better Oral Health: an evidence-based toolkit for prevention.* 2nd ed. London: The Department of Health and the British Association for the Study of Community Dentistry; 2009.

Department of Health. *The General Dental Services Statement of Financial Entitlement and the Personal Dental Services Statement of Financial Entitlement (Amendment No. 2) Directions 2011.* London: Department of Health; 2011.

Department of Health. *Health Technical Memorandum 01-05: decontamination in primary care dental practices.* 2nd ed. Leeds: Department of Health; 2013.

Department of Health. *Standards for Better Health.* London: Department of Health; 2004.

DiMatteo MR, Hays RD, Prince LM. Relationship of physicians' nonverbal communication skill to patient satisfaction, appointment noncompliance, and physician workload. *Health Psychol.* 1986; **5**(6): 581–94.

Diploma of Membership of the Joint Dental Faculties of the Royal College of Surgeons of England, MJDF Portfolio Guide 2010, version 2, MJDF available at www.mjdf.org.uk/docs/portfolio_guide.pdf

Dreyfus HL, Dreyfus SE. *Mind Over Machine: the power of human intuition and expertise in the age of the computer.* Oxford: Basil Blackwell; 1986.

Ericsson KA, Krampe R Th, Tesch-Romer C. The role of deliberate practice in the acquisition of expert performance. *Psychol Rev.* 1993; **100**: 393–4.

Faculty of General Dental Practice (UK). *Adult Antimicrobial Prescribing in Primary Dental Care for GDPs.* 2nd ed. London: FGDP (UK); 2012.

Faculty of General Dental Practice (UK). *Clinical Examination and Record-Keeping: good practice guidelines.* 2nd ed. London: Faculty of General Dental Practice (UK)'s series of standards for dental professionals; 2009.

Faculty of General Dental Practice (UK). *Key Skills in Primary Dental Care* (CD-ROM), version 2. Smile-on Ltd; 2007.

Geddes D. Travel and subsistence for dentists undertaking verifiable continuing professional development. Primary Care Commissioning Newsletter. 2013, 29 May; (5): 1–2 available at: www.england.nhs.uk/wp-content/uploads/2013/09/pc-newslt-5.pdf

General Dental Council available at: www.gdcuk.org/Membersofpublic/Lookfora specialist/Pages/default.aspx

General Dental Council. *Continuing Professional Development for Dental Professionals.* London: General Dental Council; 2013.

General Dental Council. *The First Five Years: the undergraduate dental curriculum.* 3rd ed. (interim). London: General Dental Council; 2008.

General Dental Council. *Preparing for Practice: dental team learning outcomes for registration.* London: General Dental Council; 2012.

General Dental Council. *Principles of Complaint Handling*. Reprint edition. London: General Dental Council; 2009.

General Dental Council. *Scope of Practice*. London: General Dental Council; 2013.

General Dental Council. *Standards for the Dental Team*. London: General Dental Council; 2013.

Gibbs G. *Learning by Doing: a guide to teaching and learning methods*. Oxford: Further Education Unit, Oxford Polytechnic; 1988.

Gillon R. Ethics needs principles – four can encompass the rest – and respect for autonomy should be 'first among equals'. *J Med Ethics*. 2003; **29**: 307–12.

Gilmour A, Jones R, Bullock AD. *Dental Foundation Trainers' Expectations of a Dental Graduate*. Final Report. Cardiff: Wales Deanery/Cardiff University; 2012.

Gladwell M. *Outliers: the story of success*. 1st ed. New York, NY: Little, Brown and Company; 2008.

Hemery D. *Sporting Excellence: what makes a champion?* London: Collins Willow; 1991.

Hickson GB, Clayton EW, Entman SS, *et al*. Obstetricians' prior malpractice experience and patients' satisfaction with care. *JAMA*. 1994; **272**(20): 1583–7.

Honey P, Mumford A. *Manual of Learning Styles*. London: P Honey; 1982.

Howe N, Strauss W. *Generations: the history of America's future, 1584 to 2069*. Reprint edition. New York: Perennial; 1992.

The Institute of Conservation. *Professional Standards for Conservation*. London: Institute of Conservation; 2003.

James T, Gilmour AS. Magnifying loupes in modern dental practice: an update. *Dent Update*. 2010; **37**(9): 633–6.

Kolb DA. *Experiential Learning*. Englewood Cliffs, NJ: Prentice Hall; 1984.

Krause HR, Bremerich A, Rustemeyer J. Reasons for patients' discontent and litigation. *J Craniomaxillofac Surg*. 2001; **29**(3): 181–3.

Kruger J, Dunning D. Unskilled and unaware of it: how difficulties in recognizing one's own incompetence lead to inflated self-assessments. *J Pers Soc Psychol*. 1999; **77**(6): 1121–34.

Laing & Buisson. *Dentistry UK Market Report*. London: Laing & Buisson; 2011.

Launer J. *Supervision, Mentoring and Coaching: one-to-one learning encounter in medical education*. Edinburgh: Association for the Study of Medical Education; 2006.

Lipp M, Dick W, Daubländer M, *et al*. [Different information patterns and their influence on patient anxiety before dental local anaesthesia] [German]. *Dtsch Z Mund Kiefer Gesichtschir*. 1991; **15**(6): 449–57.

London Shared Services working in partnership with COPDEND for DFT national recruitment 2014. *Nationally Coordinated Dental Foundation Training Recruitment in England, Wales and Northern Ireland 2014 Applicant Guidance, version 1*. London: London Shared Services working in partnership with COPDEND; 2013.

Lynch CD, Frazier KB, McConnell RJ, *et al*. State-of-the-art techniques in operative dentistry: contemporary teaching of posterior composites in UK and Irish dental schools. *Br Dent J*. 2010; **209**(3): 129–36.

Mangharam J, McGlothan JD. Ergonomics and Dentistry: a literature review. In: Murphy

DC, editor. *Ergonomics and the Dental Care Worker.* Washington, DC: American Public Health Association; 1998.

Mannes AE, Moore DA. A behavioral demonstration of overconfidence in judgment. *Psychol Sci.* 2013; **24**(7): 1190–7.

Miller GE. The assessment of clinical skills/competence/performance. *Acad Med.* 1990; **65**(9 Suppl.): S63–7.

Myers HL, Myers LB. 'It's difficult being a dentist': stress and health in the general dental practitioner. *Br Dent J.* 2004; **197**(2): 89–93; discussion 83; quiz 100–1.

The National Health Service (Dental Charges) Regulations 2005 (SI 2005/3477). Available at: www.legislation.gov.uk/uksi/2005/3477/schedules/made

The National Health Service (General Dental Services Contracts) Regulations 2005 (SI 2005/3361). Available at: www.legislation.gov.uk/uksi/2005/3361/regulation/2/made

The National Health Service (Performers Lists) (England) Regulations 2013 (SI 2013/335). Available at: www.legislation.gov.uk/uksi/2013/335/note/made

NHS England. *Local Professional Networks: single operating framework.* London: NHS England; 2013.

National Institute for Clinical Excellence. *Principles for Best Practice in Clinical Audit.* Oxford: Radcliffe Medical Press; 2002.

NICE Clinical Guideline 19. *Dental Recall: recall interval between routine dental examinations*; October 2004.

NICE Technology Appraisal Guidance – No.1. *Guidance on the Extraction of Wisdom Teeth*; March 2000.

Nimmons S. *Enterprise Architecture Patterns: the bold decision Maker*; 2011. Available at http://stevenimmons.org/2011/12/enterprise-architecture-patterns-the-bold-decision-maker/

Office for National Statistics. *News Release: UK population projected to hit 70m by 2027.* Office for National Statistics; 2011

Office of Fair Trading (OFT). *Dentistry: an OFT market study.* London: OFT; 2012.

O'Neill O. Some limits of informed consent. *J Med Ethics.* 2003; **29**: 4–7.

Oxford English Dictionary. Available at: www.oxforddictionaries.com/

The Personal Dental Services Statement of Financial Entitlements. Available at: www.gov.uk/

Patterson F, Ashworth V, Mehra S, *et al.* Could situational judgement tests be used for selection into dental foundation training? *Br Dent J.* 2012: **213**: 23–6.

Primary Care Contracting. *Dentists with Special Interests (DwSIs): a step by step guide to setting up a DwSI service.* London: NHS Primary Care Contracting; 2006.

Primary Care Contracting. *Primary Care Dental Services: clinical governance framework.* London: Primary Care Contracting; 2006.

Rattan R. Duty of care. *Dentist magazine.* 2011; **27**(4).

Reason J. Human error: models and management. *BMJ.* 2000; **320**: 768–70.

Resuscitation Council (UK). *Medical Emergencies and Resuscitation: standards for clinical practice and training for dental practitioners and dental care professionals in general dental practice, Revised 2012.* London: Resuscitation Council (UK); 2012.

Robinson WL. Conscious competency: the mark of a competent instructor. *Personnel Journal.* 1974; 53: 538–9.

Roethlisberger FJ, Dickson WJ. *Management and the Worker: an account of a research program conducted by the Western Electric Company. Hawthorne Works, Chicago.* Harvard University Press; 1939.

Rollnick S, Kinnersley P, Stott N. Methods of helping patients with behaviour change. *BMJ.* 1993; **307**(6897): 188–90.

Royal College of Psychiatrists. *Undertaking a Clinical Audit Project: a step-by-step guide.* Available at: www.rcpsych.ac.uk/pdf/clinauditchap2.pdf

Sancho FM, Ruiz CN. Risk of suicide amongst dentists: myth or reality? *Int Dent J.* 2010; **60**(6): 411–18.

Schön DA. *The Reflective Practitioner: how professionals think in action.* New York, NY: Basic Books; 1983.

Smithers S, Catano VM, Cunningham DP. What predicts performance in Canadian dental schools? *J Dent Educ.* 2004; **68**(6): 596–613.

Smoll FL. Effects of precision of information feedback upon acquisition of a motor skill. *Research Quarterly.* 1972; **43**: 489–93.

The Social Network. Film. Directed by Fincher D, USA. Columbia Pictures; 2010.

Sridharansend D, Levitin DJ, Chafe CH, *et al.* Neural dynamics of event segmentation in music: converging evidence for dissociable ventral and dorsal networks. *Neuron.* 2007; **55**(3): 521–32.

The Standard Clauses for a Personal Dental Services Agreement revised April 2013. Available at: www.gov.uk/government/publications/standard-general-dental-services-contract-and-personal-dental-services-agreement

The Standard General Dental Services Contract revised April 2013. Available at: www.gov.uk/government/publications/standard-general-dental-services-contract-and-personal-dental-services-agreement

Wojtczak A. Institute for International Medical Education. *Glossary of Medical Education Terms.* Available at: www.iime.org/glossary.htm

Wozniak PA, Biedalak K. The SuperMemo method: optimization of learning. *Informatyka.* 1992; 10: 1–9.

Yamalik N. Dentist-patient relationship and quality care 3. Communication. *Int Dent J.* 2005; **55**(4): 254–6.

Zhang J, Patel VL, Johnson TR. Medical error: is the solution medical or cognitive? *J Am Med Inform Assoc.* 2008; **9**(6 Suppl. 1): S75–7.

Index